Taming Your
MONSTER
Appetite

Find a Healthy Lifestyle You Can Live With

Taming Your Monster Appetite
Find a Healthy Lifestyle You Can Live With
Jennifer Minigh, PhD
Copyright @ 2018 Jennifer Minigh
ISBN: 978-0-692-11819-1

Illustrations provided by Josh Hickey. Cover photography provided by Heather May Photography. Photo of author provided by Shelby Petitt Photography. Additional photographs obtained from Fotolia.

The purpose of this book is to educate and enlighten. This book is sold with the understanding that the author and publisher are not engaged in rendering counseling, albeit it professional or lay, to the reader or anyone else. Seek the guidance of a medical physician before initiating any diet or exercise program. The author and publisher shall have neither liability nor responsibility to any person or entity with respect to any loss or damage caused, or alleged to have been caused, directly or indirectly, by the information contained in this book.

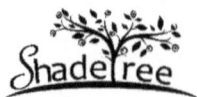

ShadeTree

CONTENTS

Introduction

Have you ever seen a kid nag someone for a piece of candy in the checkout aisle? Sometimes it's just easier for the parent to hand over the candy than it is to take a stand, especially when the same battle is repetitive and occurs often. However, if the child begged to eat lead paint chips, do you think the parent would give in? Of course not! But what if the situation was slightly changed, and it was your appetite nagging you for ice cream, despite the fact that you are already full after a large meal? Sometimes we need to separate our ravenous appetite from ourselves and treat it as a willful monster that insists on eating self-destructive stuff.

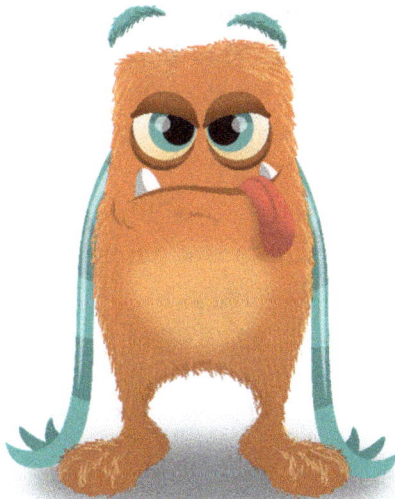

Where does this monster come from?

In reality, this monster was not always a monster. Very young children only eat when they are hungry, they have no bad eating habits, and they have absolutely no intention of sitting still. The beastly appetite for food and inactivity tends to be awakened in early childhood by parents and guardians. We demonstrate what to eat; we show them how to be picky or flexible with their food choices; we teach them what and how much is acceptable to consume; and we take away all of their recess time and force them to sit still for hours on end. All they know is what we teach and model for them; therefore, parents and guardians are the first ones who begin to foster the evolution of a normal appetite into a monstrous one. Once active, the monster feeds its own desires and grows. In the late teen and early adult years, it begins to grow unchecked, and it continues to do so until its owner intervenes.

The purpose of this book is to teach you how to tame and retrain your appetite, and your lifestyle in general, by reprogramming your mind-set about food and exercise, and by breaking your dysfunctional relationship with food.

The concepts I share in this book are not what I or my husband read from other books, but are an accumulation of our family's experiences of trial and error over the past ten years.

After reading this book, you will have:

*   an understanding of the difference between dieting and a lifestyle change;
*   an acute awareness of food quality, portion sizes, and marketing ploys to trick you;
*   an arsenal of tools to overcome hunger, temptation, and bad food choices; and
*   an appreciation for exercise and new foods.

This book was designed to be absorbed in layers, so that each time it's read it imparts additional information and inspiration at deeper and more detailed levels. We encourage you to read it multiple times to get the full benefit.

After reading the book and identifying your personal problem areas, concentrate on correcting a single issue for an entire month, or longer if needed, until you are confident that the change is permanent in your life. Don't move on to the next thing if you haven't conquered the previous one, or you'll be dealing with double the temptations and issues.

You decide which lifestyle change to make each month. Create a goal page and hang it on the fridge or somewhere very visible. Take a photo and use it for your background or wallpaper on your mobile device. Make copies and take to work or wherever else you spend time. Do whatever it takes to keep your monthly goal in the front of your mind.

Please note that what works for our family may not work for yours. Yes, we may suggest food items that have artificial sweeteners or other additives. You can decide which is worse—to eat a few additives or to continue in your current eating lifestyle, and if you're overweight, risk diabetes or heart disease, and certainly have a lower quality of life due to low energy and/or mobility.

Our fundamental goal isn't to get rid of extra weight or inactivity, but to get rid of the behaviors that cause these things. A change that will endure takes time to establish. Be patient and persevere. Just like waistlines, an appetite monster doesn't grow overnight, and likewise, it takes time to exterminate.

Taming Your Monster Appetite by Jennifer Minigh

Tame Your Mind, First

Before we can ever take on our appetite monster, we must first address its primary source of power—our thoughts.

We need to first change our mind-sets before we can be successful at changing our lifestyle. This requires us to take a hard look at our current thinking about food and fitness and make adjustments where needed.

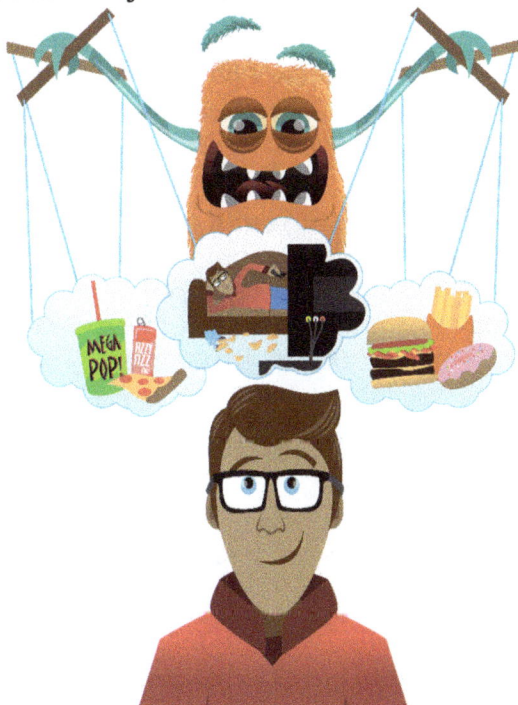

What Is Food to You?

Food is fuel for the body, like gasoline is fuel for your car. Nothing more; nothing less. However, if you ask someone to define the word *food*, you will get a plethora of responses. Do you identify with any of the following responses?

To me, food is an indication of happiness and self-control. —JOSH

****

Food is my emotional crutch. —CINDY

****

To me, it's your personality, your journey, your soul in a bowl! —JUDY

****

Fish are friends, not food. —BRUCE THE SHARK

****

My doctor told me I had to stop throwing intimate dinners for four unless there are three other people. —ORSON WELLES

****

It's easy to attach certain foods to memories of comfort and happier times. So when we are sad or miss those certain people and family, we look to eat that food and find a little comfort in it. —KIMBERLY

****

Food can be my friend or my enemy! —JERRY

****

Food is a language we all speak. It brings all races, ages, and genders together. —SHAWNDA

****

Food is communion, and good food makes for good communion. —BRANDON

PROBLEMS WITH FOOD

Food is NOT our enemy. For example, chocolate does not tempt us, but instead, we tempt ourselves with chocolate. For whatever reasons, problems with food can arise in someone's life, and when they do, action is required.

Food Addiction. When groups of food addicts and non-addicts were questioned about food addiction, six characteristics were consistently identified:[1]

1) Reward-driven eating (i.e., eating for psychological rather than physiological reasons)
2) Preoccupation with food
3) Perceived lack of self-control around food
4) Frequent food cravings
5) Increased weight or an unhealthy diet
6) Problems with specific types of food

None of these characteristics should be surprising after having read what food means to people. In today's society, food has become a means of coping, pacifying ourselves, thwarting loneliness, rewarding success, dealing with loss, etc. In order to change our lifestyle, we must change our mind-set about what food is to us, and we may even need to end some love affairs with it.

Battle of the Stomach versus Brain. Our body has two distinct nervous networks. Our central nervous system is composed of our brain and spinal cord, whereas our enteric nervous system consists of a mesh-like system of nerve cells that control the functioning of our gastrointestinal (GI) tract. This network of nerves lining our intestines is so extensive that some scientists refer to it as our second brain, or our gut brain.

This gut brain does not have conscious thoughts, but instead controls the elaborate daily grind of digestion and absorption of nutrients and has the ability to do this almost entirely independent from our head brain. In fact, for the vagus nerve (a nerve that commands unconscious body procedures, such as keeping a constant heart rate and controlling digestion), about 90 percent of the fibers carry information from the gut to the brain *and not* the other way around. Our gut brain may not make our conscience decisions; it does affect them. If you've ever "gone with your gut" when making a decision or felt butterflies in your stomach, then you're likely getting signals from your second brain.

Our head brain controls desires for food, whereas our gut brain is more aligned with controlling hunger (true hunger, not perceived hunger). In order to change our lifestyle, especially regarding food, we must work on both mind-sets and bring them into alignment instead of letting them battle each other.

The Never-ending Cycle of Dieting. A diet is a temporary change in the way one eats with the goal of losing weight. Did you catch that? "*Temporary.*" All diets come to an end in one of three ways:

#1 The person reaches the weight-loss goal and makes a conscious decision to officially end the diet.

#2 Due to a growing weariness of the diet and its restrictions, the person slowly transitions off the diet and back into the old ways of eating that caused the problem in the first place.

#3 The person never ends or completes a diet, but simply starts a new one in the middle of the previous one.

> **Jennifer Minigh**
> @jenniferminigh
>
> What's the best way to gain 10 lbs in 2 days? Plan a #diet for 3rd day. #food #foodie #weightloss

I've honestly never heard of anyone doing #1, and because dieting is a vicious cycle, #2 and #3 are the most common reasons.

I once tried the Atkin's Diet and lost thirty pounds. I've also tried diet pills and supplements. Every dieting method I've ever tried worked. That's good news, right? Well... theoretically, a person should only ever have to diet one time, because once the weight is gone, it should remain gone. But we all know, that's not how dieting works. Studies show that fewer than two out of ten individuals who lost weight were able to achieve and maintain a 10 percent reduction over the period of a year. [2] Furthermore, over one-third of the weight that was lost tended to return within the first year, and the majority was gained back within three to five years. [3,4] Dieting is a downward spiral that people get trapped in, especially since many of the diets (like ones aimed at low carbohydrates ["carbs"] or use HCG) induce changes in our natural hormones that cause disastrous rebound effects when we go off them. It's time to change your mind-set, break the cycles, and make a permanent lifestyle change that eradicates dieting forever!

QUICK FIXES

In today's click-to-make-it-happen society, quick fixes are "the bomb." Hardly anyone is willing to put time and effort into getting the results they desire. It's much more appealing to take shortcuts.

Weight-Loss Drugs. Researchers are constantly on the hunt for the magic diet pill; however, I'm convinced we have a better chance of finding the ever-elusive Bigfoot. So, what makes this search for the medicinal unicorn so difficult? After all, we've seen several weight-loss pills enter the market. What happens to them?

Many of these drugs are licensed for only a short time before being withdrawn due to unacceptable side effects. People taking the drugs often experience problems with increased blood pressure and heart rate, anxiety, depression, and suicide, as well as heart valve issues with an increased risk of pulmonary hypertension.

Another major reason for limited success is that the gut-brain system is very complex and involves many feedback mechanisms and neurotransmitters. Most weight-loss drugs are designed to target neurotransmitter systems like the serotonin, dopamine, and noradrenaline ones.

* Serotonin in the brain is thought to regulate anxiety, happiness, and mood, and low levels of it have been associated with depression.
* Dopamine helps control the brain's reward and pleasure centers (both linked with addiction), and also helps regulate movement and emotional responses; too much dopamine can induce schizophrenia, while too little can induce Parkinson's symptoms.

* Noradrenaline mobilizes the brain and body for action and is the main neurotransmitter that causes the fight-or-flight response. In the brain, noradrenaline increases alertness, enhances memory, and increases focused attention. Amphetamines (a common ingredient in diet pills) cause the release of noradrenaline, and thus is used for the treatment of narcolepsy and attention deficit disorder.

Weight-loss drugs are designed to work at these main neurotransmitter systems because of how they affect mood, appetite, and energy levels.

The enteric nervous system uses most of the same neurotransmitters the brain does. In fact, something like 95 percent of the body's serotonin is found in the bowels. This means that if you are taking a serotonin-regulating antidepressant to alter the chemicals in the brain, you may unbalance your GI system. And likewise, if you take serotonin-regulating diet pills to control hunger, you will affect the chemical balance in your brain. Irritable bowel syndrome arises in part from too much serotonin in the GI tract and is sometimes regarded as a "mental illness of the second brain."

The most probable reason that weight-loss drugs don't work is because the issues with food are generally emotional ones and not physical ones. (Remember all the emotional ties people have with food described in the introduction of this book?)

When someone takes diet pills, they risk serious health consequences, including drug addiction. A diet pill only addresses the symptoms. The real cure is a lifestyle change. It's time for folks to just say no to drugs and think outside the pill box.

Fad Diets. When I refer to "fad diets," I'm not meaning the most popular diets, like South Beach, Atkin's, Weight Watchers, or Nutrisystem. While these are all diets (as opposed to lifestyle changes) and not meant for lifetime use, they do produce results. Following are some of the fad diets to which I'm referring. Honestly, some of these are so absurd, it's hard to believe folks would even try them; however, I'm not one to judge desperation.

* The *Werewolf Diet* (also called the Lunar Diet) starts with an initial fast during the full moon, then follows a series of eating plans that change according to the phases of the moon. Yes, you may weigh less the day after the fast, but it's likely due to water loss.

* The *Baby Food Diet* requires dieters to replace breakfast and lunch with baby food, then eat a low-calorie dinner.

* The *Sleeping Beauty Diet* is based on the premise that if you're asleep, you're not eating. This diet calls for people to use sedatives to stay asleep for days on end in order to starve the body. But unfortunately, the lack of movement while on this diet causes muscle deterioration, and actually risks death.

* The *Five-Bite Diet* requires you to skip breakfast (a big no-no) and eat only five bites of food for lunch and five more bites for dinner. Later in this book we talk about eating smaller portion sizes, but this is nowhere close to what we mean. Simply put, a human body is not meant to run on this small amount of fuel, or nutrients.

* *Cookie Diets* claim that eating cookies will help you drop pounds. However, these aren't the "yummy" cookies you're hoping for. Instead, they are high-protein and high-fiber weight-loss cookies that you eat for breakfast, lunch, and snacks, followed by a low-calorie dinner. Yes, you may lose some weight, but by depriving

yourself all day, you risk bingeing at dinnertime. (Binging is *not* an eating habit we are hoping to create!)

* The *HCG Diet* mandates that you consume about 500 calories a day while taking human chorionic gonadotropin (HCG), a pregnancy hormone touted as an appetite suppressant. It's no wonder people lose weight on this diet (since they are actually existing on the edge of starvation). Furthermore, when they go off the HCG and calorie restriction, the rebound weight gain is disastrous, and many people gain far more than they ever lost. Personally, I despise this diet because I've seen the mess it has made in the lives of friends.

* The *Tapeworm Diet* is all kinds of bad. The dieter purposely ingests tapeworm eggs, then later, the hatched tapeworms consume the calories and nutrients from the dieter's eaten food. When dieters are satisfied with their weight loss (or the can't stand the side effects any longer), they ask a doctor to prescribe an anti-worm medication. Sounds nice and neat, right? I don't know about you, but there is no way I want a bunch of thirty-foot-long worms in my belly, or even worse, smaller ones escaping my intestines and making their way to other body organs—including my brain.

Trendy Gadgets. It never fails—every yard sale has at least one. You know what I mean. All those miracle-working exercise gadgets that are guaranteed to help you reach your goal weight and give you the body of a fitness model while costing you only five minutes a day. Shoes that shape your buttocks during use; a weight that you can shake back and forth; a belt that magically tones your abs while you binge-watch your new favorite series. Now, don't get me wrong. I'm not condemning all of these contraptions. Most of them work; albeit they require far more effort and time than the infomercial claimed.

Surgical Intervention. A nip and a tuck here, and a week or so of recover there—and *voilá!*—a new you. Who needs to work out for six months to get those glutes or that svelte tummy, when implants and tummy tucks are available? Cosmetic surgery can be a quick fix for weight loss and body toning.

Not all surgical interventions are cosmetic, though. One of the most successful interventions in weight loss is bariatric surgery, which includes procedures that either reduce stomach size, bypass part of the intestine, or comprise a combination of the two.

People who have these procedures lose weight at alarming speeds; nevertheless, this isn't a quick fix, as it takes months of counseling, decision-making, surgery prep, etc. Also, bariatric surgery is not entirely safe. Some of the common side effects have serious consequences and continue throughout the lifetime of the patient.

Although bariatric surgery is commonly viewed as a low-effort means of losing weight, it most certainly *is not*. Anyone who has undergone this procedure understands the effort it takes to plan and prepare meals that work afterward. Sometimes this effort is too much, and postsurgical patients resort to "easy eating" (i.e., drinking milk shakes, etc.).

Bariatric surgery often produces mixed results. While many patients initially experience massive weight loss, the results may not endure, and long-term success is highly variable—much of this is owing to the struggle with bad eating habits that persist after surgery, or other issues, like compensating for the inability to consume large volumes of food by eating dessert first so they can be sure to get it before running out of room.

When it comes to weight-loss surgery, the balance of risks versus benefits is different for each person. If you are reading this and you have experienced success with bariatric weight loss, then kudos to you! You have worked hard and sacrificed much for that success. It's important to remember that there are instances when the removal of a monster appetite needs some surgical intervention!

For those of you who know someone who is planning to have weight-loss surgery or who already has, please don't shame them or make them feel like a failure because they couldn't lose weight in other ways. They need your love, support, and encouragement for taking such a brave step to radically change their life for the better. Before people cast judgment on others, they need to ask themselves how far they would go to be healthier, or if it's even that important to them.

BUILDING NEW MIND-SETS

Even if a person undergoes a radical intervention for weight loss, like bariatric surgery, they still must embrace behavioral changes if they are to be successful. But, alas, behavioral changes are not enough, if not supported by a proper mind-set.

Listed in the beginning of this chapter are various ways that people define *food*. These ideas, in and of themselves, are not problematic. If you identified with any of them *and* you struggle with food, then you need a new mind-set.

Diane Robinson, PhD, a neuropsychologist and the program director of Integrative Medicine at Orlando Health, said:[5] "Most people focus almost entirely on the physical aspects of weight loss, like diet and exercise. But there is an emotional component to food that the vast majority of people simply overlook, and it can quickly sabotage their efforts."

The goal to creating a new mind-set about food is to take our emotions out of eating and see food as nourishment and not as a reward or a coping mechanism. An old proverb says that "as a man thinketh, so is he,"[6] meaning that we become our thoughts. If we want a new lifestyle, then we must change our thinking.

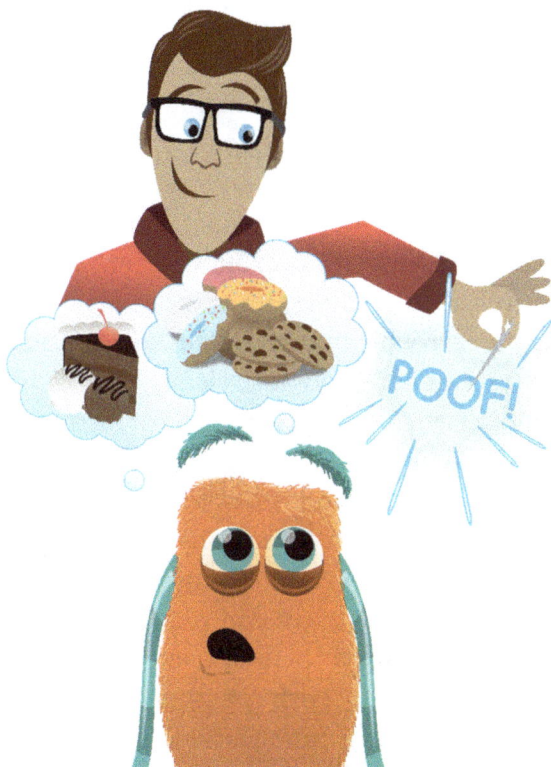

Neuroplasticity. Did you know that you can change the way you think? I'm not talking about changing your opinions about things. I'm referring to the ability of your brain to rewire itself to create new thought processes, so that old thoughts and reactions don't even come to mind, but are replaced with new ones. In the medical world, this ability for the brain to grow and rewire itself is called neuroplasticity, where *neuro* means "nerve" and *plasticity* means "the capacity for being molded or altered."

Research has shown that meditation and a focus on our thoughts can lead to actual physical brain changes. In one study,[7] brain scans from participants were obtained before and after they underwent an eight-week meditation program. The results suggest that participation in the program was associated with discernible changes in brain areas involved in learning and memory processes and emotion regulation. This is scientific evidence that when we meditate, it physically changes our brains.

By changing our thoughts, we can change our brains. So how long do such "neuroplastic" changes in the brain take to achieve? It depends on how strong the thinking is and how much it has been reinforced. For example, consider a person who has an obsessive tendency (like a constant tapping of the foot to release stress or excessive amounts of energy). This person can perform this action a thousand times a day, and every day that goes by, the habit becomes more learned and harder to overturn. Training for new things, on the other hand, shouldn't take nearly as long. In one study,[8] researchers demonstrate that forty cumulative hours of leisurely golf practice (over a range of 92 to 235 days) resulted in increased gray matter in the brain of novice golfers. Perhaps this research could be extrapolated to learning new things in general (like new lifestyle approaches) and give us an idea of how long it may take.

It is important to note that changes in the brain and how we perceive things need not be based on truths. Scientific evidence has shown that our brains have the ability to create false memories. In one study,[9] participants viewed a short film and were given a questionnaire afterward. All the questions, except one, were used as filler, while the one question asked respondents to recall a phrase that one of the characters had spoken during the film. In reality, though, that particular character *never spoke*; nevertheless, twenty-three of the thirty respondents recalled having heard him speak, and they even specifically recalled his words.

So, what does this mean for us and our pursuit for building new mind-sets? If we are not careful, we can build new mind-sets based on untruths—so it's important to be informed.

Change What We Think of Food. Somewhere along the timeline of society and culture, a shift happened. Instead of people eating to live, they began to eat. Following are some new mind-sets about food and ways to implement them.

* *Food is not a reward.* Stop celebrating successes with ice cream, favorite dinners, etc, as that will only strengthen this misconception. Instead, start using other tactics, like road trips, fresh flowers, spa treatments, or even permission to just chill out for a day as a reward.

* *Food is not a coping mechanism.* Stop using food to fill voids or induce mind-numbing trances, and start finding other ways to cope, such as meditation, reprioritizing to eliminate stress, joining a support group, volunteering, etc.

* *Food is not a requirement for being happy.* Stop equating your happiness with what you get to eat for the day. Stop allowing your happiness to be stolen if your food arrives cold, burnt, late, or not exactly as you ordered it. Resolve to be content, despite your circumstances.

* *Stop believing that only good-tasting food can be eaten.* Try to be more tolerant of less-desirable foods. Be open to trying new foods that are healthy. Because some tastes must be acquired, every few months, try a new healthy food that you currently don't like; eventually, you will learn to like it. Don't try new foods that are bad choices so that you avoid developing a love for it. Better

to never know what something tastes like than to constantly have to fend off cravings for it.

*   *Food is not a companion.* If you have a love affair with food, then break it off. And for goodness' sake, stop taking selfies with it like it's your best buddy! Limit how often you eat alone.

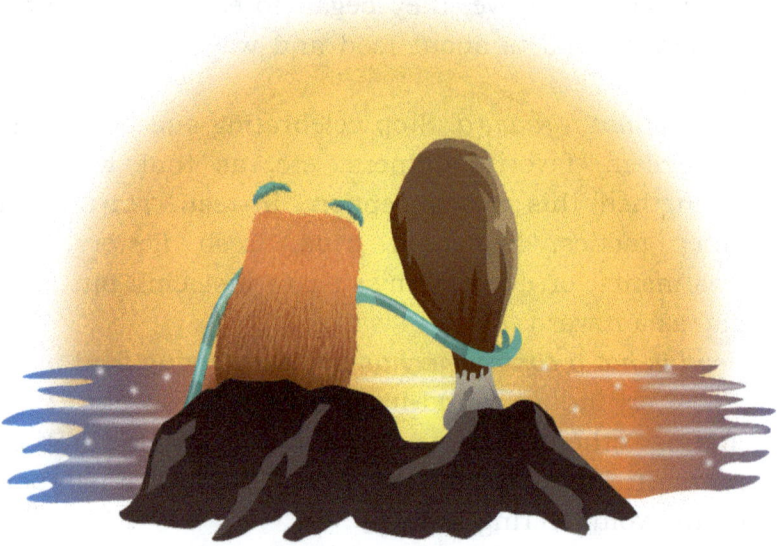

*   *Food is not a requirement for social gatherings.* Research shows that food tastes better when eaten with company, even when the company is just yourself in the mirror. [10] Food is a large component of social gatherings and often considered social glue. Instead of doing away with food at events altogether, though, add some social gatherings into your calendar that don't incorporate food. For example, have a bowling night with a group of friends, but don't eat as a group before, during, or after it. Don't do away with all food-related events; just add some balance. If food is a must for an event, challenge everyone to bring something healthy, along with the recipe to share.

When we change the way we think about food and we develop healthy mind-sets about it, our lifestyle choices will fall in line. Consider the following testimonies:

> *After eating healthy for over six years, I only crave the stuff I can eat. Your snacks are safe around me, because I just don't see them as food for me.* —LYNN

****

Today's food is tomorrow's energy. —JOHN

Change What We Think about Our Bodies. Body image is a huge problem, especially for many women. Here are some new mind-sets to adopt about our bodies.

* *Our bodies are tools for us.* Just like astronauts need a special suit in order to live in outer space, we (who are spirit beings) need a "dirt suit" (a physical body) to live on the earth. Our body is a tool for our spirit to get around and function within the physical realm of the earth.

* *Our bodies are under our jurisdiction and control.* Just like with our cars, we drive our bodies, and they don't drive us. When you sit in the driver's seat of a car, the steering wheel doesn't latch on to your hands and turn them in the direction of your travel. *You* control the car. The same is true for your body.

* *Our brains are like the managers of our bodies.* Think of your brain as a manager who carries out your requests and who minds the shop (like keeping your heart beating and your lungs breathing) when you're preoccupied with other missions. If you instruct your body to take three steps forward, the brain (your manager) sets all the workers (like the nerves, muscles, etc.) into motion, and your legs comply and take the steps you wanted to take.

* *Our brains can be rewired to think new thoughts and respond in new ways.* Just like when a new task comes up at your job and everyone needs training to learn to do it, sometimes you will need to train your brain to respond in new ways. This requires constant and vigilant monitoring of all incoming thoughts. Every thought must be captured and weighed against the new standards you are setting. If the thought does not line up with the new mind-set, or if it introduces conflicting streams of thought, it must be cast down and destroyed immediately.

* *Our bodies provide important feedback to us.* The relationship you have with your brain and your body goes both ways. For example, once your body becomes accustomed to eating only healthy foods, it will respond negatively when you eat something unhealthy. Adverse reactions like nausea and diarrhea are the body's way of letting you know you have made some bad choices. Theresa, a friend of mine, had been eating really well for several weeks. One day at work, the kitchen staff prepared a new soup. Despite the warnings from her inner self about the quality of the soup, she tried a single spoonful, only to have her stomach immediately start gurgling its disapproval. She couldn't believe how after only a few weeks of healthy eating, her body had so radically changed its response to foods, and it actually gave her instant feedback about her bad choice.

* *Our bodies will learn to comply with our instructions.* Sometimes we need to lead a child to the understanding that we, as the parent, know what's best, and then they come into alignment with what is acceptable and permissible. For example, as a child, I never wanted to

go to bed when I was told to; however, when we moved to a community that had a 9 p.m. curfew every evening, announced by a fire whistle, my mother declared the whistle to be my new bedtime signal. I immediately came into alignment and rarely struggled with her about bedtime after that. Once kids realize that things will be a certain way and that there is no room for variance, they begin to comply. The same is true with our bodies. If you smell bacon frying and your body tries to suggest that it is hungry (which is inappropriate, since you ate only an hour ago!), you can tell your body to stop the false feeling, and it should comply; maybe not at first, but it will with your persistent instruction. Some people call this "mind over matter," while others may think it's a big bag of hooey; however, research continues to prove that it's real, especially in terms of pain research.

When we change the way we think about our bodies and realize that they are actually magnificent machines we control ourselves, we can step into a leadership role and take authority over it—and our feelings.

Change What We Think of Fitness. Although most of this chapter until now has been about food, fitness cannot be overlooked. In our culture, the word *fitness* is tightly linked to exercise; however, fitness means so much more. The word *fit* means "the capacity of a living thing to survive and reproduce." *Physical fitness*, according to the Centers for Disease Control and Prevention (CDC) is "the ability to carry out daily tasks with vigor and alertness, without undue fatigue, and with ample energy to enjoy leisure-time pursuits and respond to emergencies."[11]

Following are some great mind-sets to hold about fitness:

It's mind, body, and spirit. —RENEE

****

Fitness undoes the unhealthy lifestyle and damage that we do to our bodies on a daily basis. —DEBBIE

****

Fitness is intentionally taking time to live a healthy lifestyle. —JILLIAN

****

Fitness is a discipline, and those who are disciplined achieve results. —AARON

****

Fitness is challenging but rewarding. —CRISTIE

****

Fitness is a healthy addiction. —NEMO

****

Fitness to me is stress relief. —DEVYN

****

Fitness is the war I wage against my doubts and lethargy. —ADAM

****

Fitness is being fit enough to live your life to its fullest potential. —ALAN

When we change the way we think about fitness, we can put our lethargic lifestyle to rest.

START TODAY!

Get rid of stinkin' thinkin' that plagues your efforts to live a healthier life. Stop letting the appetite monster control your thoughts.

Don't Wait Any Longer. You can't accomplish what you never start. When people on their deathbeds are asked about the lives they have lived, more often than not, their regrets are about what they *didn't* do and the opportunities they missed. Don't wait for a death sentence to put your perspective in order. Grab hold of a better way of thinking today, and don't let another moment escape you forever.

> **Jennifer Minigh**
> @jenniferminigh
>
> You can't accomplish what you never start.
>
> #motivation #fitness #health #wellness

Just Jump In. What is the best way to enter a cold pool on a hot day? Well, it's not by easing into it slowly—talk about prolonging the agony! Unless you can't swim, taking a giant leap into the deep end is by far the best way, because instead of fretting about how cold the water is, you focus on not drowning. Yes, the initial shock is breathtaking, but it's short-lived, and by the time you take a couple of strokes to right yourself, you're already acclimated to the temperature.

When we are expecting to endure something that we perceive as dreadful, we generally take one of three approaches. The easiest approach (and the way out) is straight-up avoidance. For example, I can't count the times I've dipped my toe into chilly water and decided that in no certain terms would I ever consider swimming in that pool, that day or maybe even ever again. Another approach is perpetual procrastination. In other words, I would stay stuck in the planning mode, and never initiate anything. I would guess that cleaning closets falls into this category for many folks. The third approach is to set an actual start date and prepare for it. However, when we have ample time to wallow in the dread of the looming event, we tend to compensate and try to make up for our pending hardship. For example, how many times have you decided to start a diet on Monday and then compensate for your perceived future deprivation by spending the whole weekend eating all your soon-to-be forbidden favorites? In situations like these, it's better to jump right in and get started.

Jennifer Minigh
@jenniferminigh

A twist on an old adage:

Why put on today, the weight you'll have to work off tomorrow...

#changeisgood #nutrition #fitness

Be Patient and Persistent. Building new mind-sets takes time. A new habit can take several weeks or months to develop. In a scientific study designed to evaluate habits,[12] participants chose one new habit to implement. Examples of the behaviors chosen were "drinking a bottle of water with lunch," or something more difficult, like "running for fifteen minutes before dinner." (There was no reward for completing the task.) Each day for twelve weeks, the participants reported whether or not they did the behavior and how "automatic" it felt. The researchers then determined how many days it took before the behavior became nearly habitual to the participants. The average time was sixty-six days, but the range was from eighteen to 254 days. (It's worth pointing out, again, that whether it takes eighteen days or 254 days, the only way to get to Day 254 is to start with Day 1!) Additional research[13] (as well as life experience) shows that behavior change is initially a *mental effort*, but the more we do it, the more natural and easier it becomes. We need only to be patient and persistent.

Start Small and Take Small Steps. Choose easier things to address first, and then build momentum that will give you the fortitude to conquer the harder ones. Choose goals that are small and manageable. For example, don't set your goal as to "lose weight," because that's too broad and overwhelming. Instead, make a list of mind-sets and habits you want to change in order to realize a healthier weight. Make the list very specific and load each item with appropriate context in which to perform the action. The context can be any cue, such as an event ("when I get home from work") or a time of day ("after breakfast"). Pick cues that are common in your daily life so that you will be required to perform the goal frequently and consistently.

Include on your list any items associated with food. For example:

* When I experience a craving for candy, I will immediately separate myself physically from its presence and not seek to obtain it.
* When I shop at the grocery store, I will not bring home chips or candy.

Include items associated with exercise. For example:

* I will set aside five minutes before my midmorning coffee to do some jumping jacks and push-ups.

* When brushing my teeth each morning, I will do squats the entire time that I am brushing.

Include items associated with negative thoughts and self-doubt. For example:

* When something upsets me, I will discharge the emotions with a brisk walk instead of reaching for food.
* When I begin to doubt myself, I will list at least ten accomplishments that I have achieved in the past week.

When you make your list of goals, choose only one in each category to work on for a day, week, or month. Don't try to address the entire list at once, as this is a surefire way to overwhelm yourself and ultimately fail before you even get started. As you successfully incorporate each goal into your life, give yourself a star beside it and pick up a new goal to work on. Start small, take small steps, and experience big successes.

Remind Yourself. Change is hard, and I'm convinced that only babies in dirty diapers like it. Make a list of the reasons you want a new lifestyle and a new way of thinking. Focus on these motives and remind yourself why you are making such wonderful efforts. Remind yourself of how much better you will feel—physically, mentally, and emotionally. Remind yourself of all of the benefits of a new lifestyle.

Be Realistic. Set reasonable and achievable goals and give yourself permission to mess up sometimes—perfection is unobtainable, and the pursuit of it only hinders our efforts to better ourselves. Take responsibility for any previous unhealthy habits and ways of thinking that may have shaped your life up to this point. Forgive yourself for them. Let go of any shame, guilt, and thoughts that you may have tried to erase with food in the past. If any issue is bigger than your ability to address, realize that you may need professional help—and don't be afraid to seek it out. Learn to discern what is real and what is merely your emotions and recognize when the monster is trying to control your thoughts.

Taming Your Monster Appetite by Jennifer Minigh

Taming Your Monster Appetite by Jennifer Minigh

Then, Mind Over Monster

Contrary to the assertion of Barbara Johnson (an American literary critic) and probably the opinion of Cookie Monster himself, a balanced diet is *not* a cookie in each hand!

In order to change our lifestyles, some education and increased awareness needs to take place, especially concerning food, fitness, and what it means to be healthy. Keeping our head stuck in the sand will not help our endeavors, and neither will allow the monster to sow corrupt thoughts, like, *If I don't know it's wrong, then is it really wrong?* Or thoughts like, *If I don't know it's bad, then I won't feel guilty for eating it.* The fact is that what we don't know *can* hurt us!

Knowledge is the power behind our ability to tame our monster appetite. We must rip off the blinders and exert our mind over the monster.

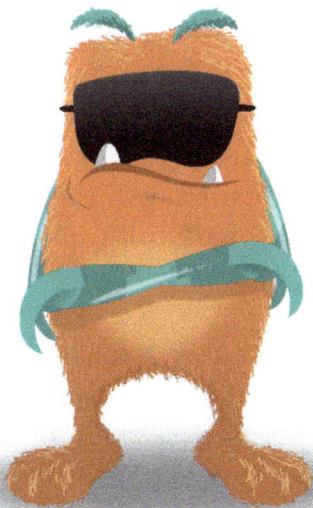

THE NEED FOR AWARENESS

In a study in Switzerland,[14] two groups of participants were presented with a buffet of 179 different foods that were common in Swiss culture. The control group was instructed to serve themselves food they would eat on a normal day, and the healthy group was told to choose food representing a healthy diet. The goal of the study was to see how consumers defined healthy food choices. The results led the researchers to conclude that, in general, people lacked any real knowledge about portion sizes and important nutrients in foods.

When you increase your awareness and understanding about food, it changes your perspective about eating, and the research proves this to be true.

> **Jennifer Minigh**
> @jenniferminigh
>
> .evitcepsrep tuoba lla s'tI
>
> Sometimes we just need to see it from a different point of view.

In a study of undergraduate women,[15] those who were trained to direct their attention toward pictures of healthy food ate more healthy snacks, compared with the women who were trained to look at pictures of unhealthy food. This research tells us that our lifestyles will follow whatever we train ourselves to prefer.

In two additional studies, researchers tested whether healthy eating habits would protect people against the temptation of consuming large portion sizes and unhealthy foods.[16] In both studies, the answer was *YES!* In the first study, participants who were trained with unhealthy habits gave in to temptation and ate more chocolate than those who were trained with healthy habits. The second study showed that participants who were trained to choose carrots as a response to seeing a certain picture subsequently resisted chocolate-covered candies as long as that picture was present. This research shows how powerful habits are, and how we can create new ones to retrain our eating lifestyles.

As we grow in our awareness and understanding of food, it will become obvious that not everyone is on the same page, or maybe even the same planet! Almost twenty years ago, David and I took our first step toward eating healthy food, when we decided to eat chicken strips instead of cheeseburgers with our fries at our favorite fast-food place. This was a huge step for us, and it felt like a tremendous sacrifice. We wallowed in our misery during each meal where we made that choice, but we also failed more often than not. One day, while working out at the local YMCA, David struck up a conversation with an older gentleman who had the body of a man decades younger. The man proceeded to explain how his impressive physique was due more to healthy eating over the years than to excessive exercise. Inspired by the gentleman's advice, David began to boast how he also "ate healthy," and then he shared how he had begun to choose chicken strips over cheeseburgers. The man, who now expressed his strong aversion for fried foods, was *appalled* at how David thought that fried chicken strips and French fries could ever be construed as "healthy food." (GASP!) Clearly the two men were not on the same page!

As you begin your journey toward a better lifestyle, just remember there are people ahead of you, and also behind you. Try to not cast judgment on either of them. We are all in this thing together, and we will continue to learn more with each passing day.

AWARENESS ABOUT FOOD QUALITY

Food for our bodies is like gas for our cars. The better gas you put in your vehicle, the better your car will run. We put the correct gas in for what our cars require. We don't add dirt or any other contaminants. Remember the days when pranksters would pour sugar into the gas tanks of their enemies? What happened to those cars? Sugar doesn't instantly kill the engine, like popular belief holds that it does, but it *will* cause problems with the way the car runs until the system is purged of it. And the owner has to take extra measures to remove the sugar. Sometimes we need to remove contaminants from our fuel so that our bodies will start to run like they were meant to.

Kitava is a tiny island off the eastern coast of Papau New Guinea in the Pacific. The two thousand or so people on the island live simple lives of fishermen, that lack the eating habits and sedentary lifestyles of many people in the Western world. The people there mainly eat coconuts, fish, tubers (i.e., potatoes), and tropical fruit. So, what is so cool about these islanders? When they were studied by researchers, not a single Kitavan who was examined had acne. [17] Not one pimple was detected—not even in the island's adolescents. These people provided a clear picture of what clean and healthy living could look like.

The quickest way to learn about the quality of your food is to read labels. Ignore all the healthy claims and advertising on the packages and go for the real truth. A food is not healthy just because its manufacturer says so.

As you visit various restaurants, you will notice that more and more are listing the calories of their meals on their menus. As you visit each place, either in person or online, make a mental list of options that fit into your lifestyle goals. This way, when you're planning to eat out, you will already know a few healthy options for each place. Focus on all the options you *can* eat instead of agonizing over what you shouldn't.

Details about the nutrient content of foods (even for specific brands) are available in the United States Department of Agriculture (USDA) Food Composition Databases at https://ndb.nal.usda.gov/ndb/search/list. I strongly encourage you to visit this Web site and browse the most common foods you eat. You can even search by restaurant in the "manufacturer" tab.

Judging Calories. (Note: For the sake of convenience in this book, the word *calorie* is used instead of the more technically correct *kilocalorie*.) The quality of food is judged by its ability to provide nutrients without a high cost of calories. If you ask folks to list the basic components of food, most people list them just like they are listed on the nutrition labels of food.

calories

carbs

protein

fat

However, calories are not in the same category as these other components. When the body burns fat, carbs, and protein, it generates calories of energy for the body to use as fuel. Instead, the list should look like this:

carbs

protein

+   fat

_____

calories

If you wanted to decrease the calories you consume, you would have a choice of decreasing the amount of fat, carbs, or protein you consume. A decrease in any of these three will result in fewer calories for the day. So, which one is the best to decrease? Consider these facts:

A gram of carbs is about **4** calories.

A gram of protein is about **4** calories.

A gram of fat is about **9** calories.

If you have studied nutrition before, then you may remember this as the 4-4-9 Rule. Just looking at these three choices, which one contributes the most calories to your intake? Yes, it's the fat. Therefore, cutting fat from your diet will reduce your calories twice as fast as cutting carbs or protein from it. Now let's consider a real-life example.

Regular peanut butter has the following general nutrition:

Regular Peanut Butter

Carbs 8 g

Protein 7 g

+   Fat 16 g
_____

Calories 190

A healthy alternative to regular peanut butter is powdered peanut butter. It is a higher-quality food.

Regular Peanut Butter	Powdered Peanut Butter
Carbs 8 g	Carbs 4 g
Protein 7 g	Protein 6 g
+ Fat 16 g	+ Fat 1.5 g
Calories 190	Calories 50

Now, let's say that twin brothers who are exactly the same size are both on a diet, and all they get is

1,500 calories to eat a day. Because they are still paying their student loans, the only thing they can afford to eat is peanut butter and jelly sandwiches. Bob makes his sandwiches with real peanut butter, while his brother, Larry, makes his with peanut butter powder.

Bob's Sandwich	Larry's Sandwich
Carbs 47 g	Carbs 41 g
Protein 11 g	Protein 10 g
+ Fat 17.5 g	+ Fat 3 g
Calories 370	Calories 230

If each one of Bob's sandwiches is 370 calories, then he can eat four sandwiches to stay under his 1,500-calorie goal. However, because Larry's sandwich was only 230 calories, he can eat six and a half sandwiches. Both men eat the exact same type of sandwich and the same number of calories, but which one will be hungrier at the end of the day? Bob will be hungrier, because he has to eat less. Larry gets to eat two and a half more sandwiches than Bob.

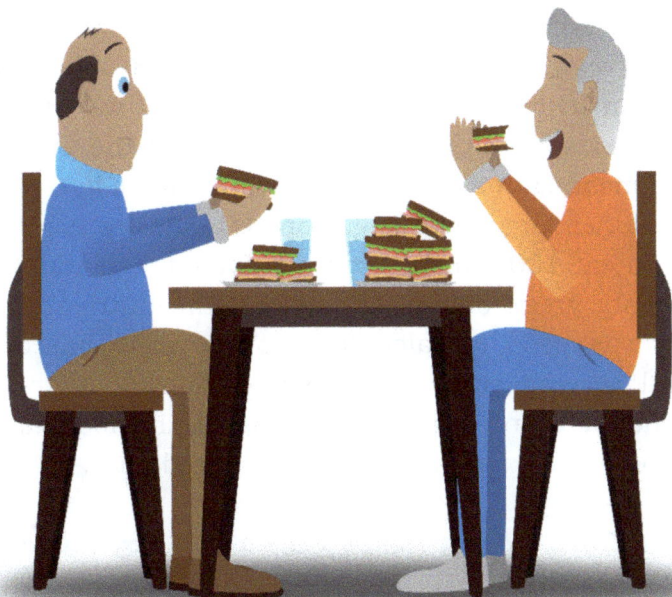

This is an example of how someone who eats high-quality food can eat more of it and be satisfied. Someone who is trying to watch his calories without limiting his fat will likely fail, due to constant and nagging hunger from not having enough to eat.

Eating foods that are higher quality requires that we become aware of what those foods are, and which foods won't fit the bill.

Judging Fruits and Vegetables. The CDC ranked forty-one powerhouse fruits and vegetables that are strongly associated with a reduced risk of chronic disease.[18] For each food, seventeen nutrients were assessed: potassium, fiber, protein, calcium, iron, thiamin, riboflavin, niacin, folate, zinc, and vitamins A, B6, B12, C, D, E, and K. A nutrient density score was calculated for each food and the nutritional profile of the food per 100 calories of it. These scores are available at this Web site: https://www.cdc.gov/pcd/issues/2014/13_0390.htm.

The nutrient density scores from the CDC were based on 100 calories of the food, and for some of the foods, this would mean eating unfathomable amounts of it, due to the low calories they have (e.g., for 100 calories, you would need to eat 100 radishes, twenty-five cups of watercress, or twenty green onions). Therefore, the nutrient density score was used to calculate another score based on a typical serving size of the food. Following is this new nutritional score per each serving of the food and the ranking of each fruit and vegetable based on it.

Top 20 Powerhouse Fruits and Vegetables

Rank	Fruit or Vegetable	Nutritional Score
1	Red pepper	19.0
2	Brussels sprouts	18.0
3	Kale	16.2
4	Parsley	14.4
5	Sweet potato	12.0
6	Carrots	11.8
7	Dandelion greens	11.6
8	Lemon	11.4
9	Turnip greens	11.2
10	Broccoli	10.8
11	Leaf lettuce	10.6
12	Pumpkin	10.1
13	Kohlrabi	9.3
14	Mustard greens	9.2
15	Chinese cabbage	9.2
16	Winter squash	8.8
17	Strawberry	8.6
18	Grapefruit (pink & red)	8.0
19	Orange	8.0
20	Grapefruit (white)	7.7

Nutritional score = (nutrient density score from the CDC)/100 X (calories per serving). Serving size = 1 cup.
https://www.cdc.gov/pcd/issues/2014/13_0390.htm

Judging Carbohydrates and Sweeteners. Carbs provide the major source of energy we need, and they are made up of three components: fiber, starch, and sugar. Fiber and starch are complex carbs, while sugar is a simple carb.

Simple carbs are found in milk, fruit, and refined sugar. Complex carbs are found in grain products such as bread, crackers, pasta, and rice. Fiber is not absorbed in the body (and therefore, it contains no calories), and it acts like a broom to sweep toxins and leftover food particles out of our intestines. Good sources of fiber include legumes, whole grains, vegetables, and fruit.

Simple carbs provide for immediate energy needs, whereas complex carbs serve as long-term energy sustainment throughout the day. Complex carbs have a lower glycemic index, meaning that you will get lower amounts of sugars released at a more consistent rate throughout the day, as opposed to peaking and crashing as you would with simple carbs.

A sweetener is anything added to a food substance in order to make the taste sweeter. A sweetener may or may not be a carbohydrate, but it makes a food substance taste like it contains carbs. Sweeteners can be either natural (whole food or extract) or artificial.

Glycemic Index. The glycemic index is a measure of how a carbohydrate-containing food raises a person's blood glucose level (also called blood sugar) two hours after the consumption of the food, and it was first developed as a tool for guiding the food choices for people with diabetes. Glycemic index values are determined experimentally by feeding a test subject a fixed amount of the food that contains 50 grams of digestible carbohydrates, and then by taking blood samples at specific intervals of time after the meal to measure the amount of glucose in the blood.

The glycemic index goes from zero to 100. For some general comparisons, glucose has a glycemic index of 100 and sucrose (table sugar) has a glycemic index of 65. Sugar alcohols have an index of zero to 3, whereas artificial sweeteners have a zero.

So, exactly what does the glycemic index tell us? Consider plums and grapes, for example. A plum has a glycemic index of 24. This means that if you eat enough plums to consume 50 grams of digestible carbohydrates, your blood glucose level after eating the plum will be 24 percent of the blood glucose level after eating the same amount of pure glucose. Compare this to eating grapes, which has a glycemic index of 49 and would result in percentage of 49. If a person with diabetes had to choose between eating plums or grapes based on glycemic index, which would be their best choice? Yes, it would be the plum, because the grapes would raise the blood sugar twice as much (i.e., 49 percent versus 24 percent).

The glycemic index is useful for more than just people with diabetes. Many popular commercial diets (e.g, the Zone Diet and Atkin's Diet) are based on carbohydrate restrictions and employ the glycemic index as a basis for choosing which carbohydrates are best to consume or restrict. Not only do low glycemic index foods decrease the body's sensitivity to insulin and improve diabetes control, they also reduce hunger, prolong physical endurance, minimize cravings, and minimize energy crashes.

One limitation of the glycemic index is that it does not reflect the likely amount you would eat for a particular food, or the fact that some foods contain more digestible carbohydrates than others. The glycemic index value is based on the *amount of digestible carbohydrate in 50 grams of the food*, but we know that different foods have different amounts of digestible carbohydrates, some having way more than others. For example, let's compare two snacks we could choose from, either one serving of watermelon or one serving of chocolate toaster pastries. Both foods have a glycemic index of about 71 (so would appear to be equally bad for us); however, each food has a different amount of digestible carbohydrates (the watermelon has 6 grams per serving and the pastry has 37 grams per serving). For these two foods to be equivalent in terms of glycemic index, we would have to eat a lot more watermelon to get to 50 grams of digestible carbohydrates than we would have to eat of the pastry. To address this problem, researchers have developed another tool, called glycemic load, which indicates changes in blood glucose when you eat a *typical serving* of the food. Determining the glycemic load involves multiplying the glycemic index by the amount of digestible carbohydrates (total carbs minus fiber) in the food and then divide by 100. Low (good) glycemic load is 1 to 10, medium is 11 to 19, and high (bad) is 20 or more.

Because the glycemic index makes watermelon and chocolate toaster pastries look equally bad for us, let's use glycemic load to compare them instead. A typical serving of diced watermelon (i.e., about a cup) has a glycemic load value of 4, which classifies it as a healthy food choice. A typical serving of chocolate toaster pastries (i.e., 1 pastry) has a glycemic load value of 26, which classifies it as an unhealthy food choice. We have a winner now. Watermelon will be our snack!

Watermelon versus a Toaster Pastry

1 serving of watermelon	1 serving of toaster pastry

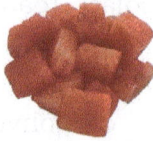

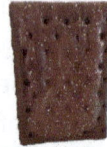

glycemic index = 71   glycemic index = 71

With GI = 71, they appear to be equally bad, BUT...

1 serving has **6 grams** of digestible carbohydrates,	1 serving has **36 grams** of digestible carbohydrates,

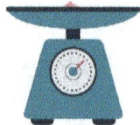

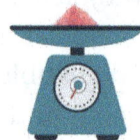

so **glycemic load = 4**   so **glycemic load = 26**
classified as   classified as
HEALTHY   **UNHEALTHY**

CONCLUSION:
The foods are **not** equal as they first appeared.
The watermelon is the healthier choice!

If glycemic index and glycemic load sound the same, and the math is downright confusing to you, then know that you're not alone! You can boil it all down to this... when you look at the amount of carbs in a food, if most of them come from sugar instead of fiber, then it's not a good choice. Instead, opt for foods that have most of the carbs coming from fiber.

An international table of glycemic index and glycemic load values for foods is available here: http://ajcn.nutrition.org/content/76/1/5/T1.expansion. html. The table contains nearly 1,300 data entries representing more than 750 different types of foods.[19] An international glycemic index database (including glycemic load measures also) is maintained by Sydney University Glycemic Index Research Services and is available here: http://www.glycemicindex.com.

Types of Sweeteners. Sweeteners come in all sorts of varieties and include whole-food natural sweeteners, natural sweeteners extracted from whole foods, and artificial sweeteners. For additional details about sweeteners, see the following table.

Types of Sweeteners

Whole-Food Natural Sweeteners
• Include honey, maple syrup, coconut palm sugar, and sorghum.
• Contain sugars in addition to other nutritive contents. Tend to have a lower glycemic index than sugars, but still need to be consumed in moderation.
Natural Sweeteners Extracted from Whole Foods
Sugars
• Include glucose, sucrose (table sugar), fructose (fruit sugar), dextrose (which is glucose and fructose bound together), maltose (malt sugar), and galactose and lactose (milk sugars).
• Provide about 4 calories per gram and have a high glycemic index.
Modified Sugars
• Produced by converting starch to sugar using enzymes.
• Often used in cooking or in processed foods and include high fructose corn syrup, refiners syrup, caramel, inverted sugar, and golden syrup.
• Provide about 4 calories per gram and have a high glycemic index.

Sugar Alcohols

- Low-digestible carbohydrates, which occur naturally in fruits, vegetables, mushrooms, etc.
- Xylitol is perhaps the most popular due to its similarity to sucrose; other sugar alcohols include sorbitol, maltitol, mannitol, erythritol, isomalt, and lactitol.
- Provide about 3 calories per gram, but have a low glycemic index.

Stevia

- Extracted from the leaves of the plant species *Stevia rebaudiana*.
- Brand names include Truvia®, Stevia In The Raw®, and PureVia®.

Thaumatin

- A sweet protein extracted from the katemfe fruit.

Artificial Sweeteners

Although many artificial sweeteners are available, this section discusses only the most widely used ones in the United States.

Aspartame

- Brand names include Equal® and Nutrasweet®.
- It has been the subject of controversy regarding its safety since its initial approval by the United States Food and Drug Administration in 1974.[20]

Acesulfame—k (potassium acesulfamate)

- Brand names include Sunett® and Sweet One®.

Sucralose

- Brand names include Splenda®, Zerocal, Sukrana®, SucraPlus, and Nevella®.

Saccharin

- Brand names include Sweet'n Low®, Necta Sweet®, Sugar Twin®, and Sweet 10®.
- In the 1970s, studies in rats suggested an association between high doses of saccharin and the development of bladder cancer.[21] As a result, the FDA mandated a label warning, which was later dropped in 2000 following new research showing that humans react differently than rats and were not at risk of cancer at typical intake levels.

Judging Proteins. Proteins provide our bodies with the building blocks they need to grow and repair tissues such as muscles, bones, blood, and organs. They are made up of amino acids. There are twenty different amino acids found within the body; eleven can be made by the body, while nine are considered essential (lysine, threonine, valine, isoleucine, leucine, methionine, phenylalanine, tryptophan, and histidine) and must be obtained through diet. The best sources of protein are poultry, fish, eggs, low-fat dairy products, nuts, seeds, and legumes like black beans and lentils.

The quality of a protein is determined by its amino acid composition and its ability to be digested and absorbed into the bloodstream. Following are two measures for protein quality.

* *Biological Value* is a measure of how much of the protein consumed is actually digested, absorbed, and used by the body. When BV was first instituted, eggs were given the highest value (i.e., 100) because they are the most bioavailable natural protein. Later, whey isolated from milk was shown to have a higher BV (104 to 154, depending on the extraction process).
* The *Protein Digestibility Corrected Amino Acid Score* is considered the gold standard for protein quality and is based not only on our ability to digest and absorb the protein, but also on the amount of essential amino acids it contains.

Sources of dietary protein are generally classified as either being of animal or vegetable origin. Animal sources of protein contain all the essential amino acids, whereas vegetable sources generally lack one or more. Furthermore, because plant cells have cell walls, it takes more energy for our bodies to digest the plant material in order to get to the proteins.

Carbohydrates and fats can be stored in the body for future use, unlike amino acids, which are excreted. This is an important consideration, because when we consume foods that contain low-BV proteins, then most of the protein will be excreted instead of used, and it will be like we didn't each much protein at all. When you are deciding to add some protein to your day, don't just pick the food with the highest amount of protein, but consider the BV values and what you are needing the protein to do for you.

Avoid foods with low-BV proteins and strive to consume foods with high values instead. Because high-BV proteins are easily absorbed by the body, they are great to consume immediately upon waking (when you are still in a fasting state from sleeping overnight) or following vigorous activity (when your body is depleted of nutrients). Foods with high-BV protein are great for people on calorie-restricted diets because the higher quality of the protein means you can eat a lower quantity of the food to get the same effect. Use the table below to decide which protein sources are best for you (important things to consider are the total protein amount, the BV, and the fat content). Also remember that protein absorption is decreased in people who have had gastric bypass surgery.

Quality of Common Protein Sources

Protein Source	Biological Value	Protein (gram)	Fat (gram)	Calories
Egg, whole (1 large, boiled)	100	6	5	78
Egg, white only (1 large, cooked)	88	6	0.4	17
Milk, whole (1 cup)	91	10	8	149
Milk, skim (1 cup)	91	10	0.6	101
Shrimp (3 oz, cooked)	90+	20	0.2	84
Cottage cheese (2% milkfat, 4 oz)	84	12	3	92
Salmon (3 oz, cooked)	83	17	5	121
Tuna, canned (in water, 3.0 oz)	83	17	1	73
Pork chop (lean, 3 oz, broiled)	82	24	5	144
Bacon (3 slices fried)	82	12	12	162
Sirloin steak (lean, 3 oz, broiled)	80	25	8	180
Venison, ground (3 oz, cooked)	80	22	7	159
Chicken breast (3 oz, grilled)	79	26	3	128
Turkey breast (3 oz, roasted)	79	26	2	125
Tofu, firm (½ cup, raw)	74	22	11	181
Peanuts (1 oz)	68	7	14	161
Almonds, sliced (¼ cup)	66	5	11	133
Kidney beans (¼ cup)	50	11	0.4	153

Many professional athletes use protein powder supplements to reach higher protein goals for their daily nutrition, in order to maintain and build more muscle mass. These supplements often contain milk protein (such as whey protein and casein), soy protein, or egg protein as their main ingredient.

While all of these proteins share excellent essential amino acid profiles, egg protein (BV 100) and whey protein (concentrate BV 104 and isolate BV 159) appear to be better used by the body then casein protein (BV 77) or soy protein (BV 74). The downsides of high-BV protein, as are included in these supplements, is that the protein is broken down quickly in the body and excreted before it can ever be used.

Judging Fats. Fats are organic molecules made up of carbon and hydrogen atoms joined together in long chains called hydrocarbons. They are the building blocks for vitamin D and hormones, and they help you to absorb vitamins A, D, E, and K. Fats are used to build and maintain brain and nerve tissue, and they are stored in your fat cells to provide insulation for the body and a long-term reservoir of energy.

Fats are classified by the type of carbon-to-carbon bonds in the fat molecule. The three main types of fat are saturated, monounsaturated, and polyunsaturated. Unsaturated fat is found in plants and fish and is mostly liquid at room temperature. Saturated fat is found in milk, meat, and processed food and is mostly solid at room temperature. Trans-fat is the unhealthiest fat and is found in most processed, baked, and fried foods. It is also found in margarine in the stick form (tub and squeeze varieties have less, so look for trans-fat–free margarines).

Seeds and nuts are high in fat because they must contain enough energy to start a new life. The same principle is true for egg yolks. In general, any plant part that is responsible for the propagation of life, or any animal part that requires high amounts of energy for use (i.e., muscle and liver) will be high in fat content.

The body can synthesize most of the fats it needs; however, two essential fatty acids (linoleic acid and alphalinolenic) cannot be made by the body, and therefore they must be obtained from food. These two essential fats are used to build omega-3 and omega-6 fatty acids, which are important for the normal functioning of tissues in the body.

Both omega-3 and omega-6 fats are derived from linoleic acid. Most diets provide adequate amounts of omega-6 fat, which is found in leafy vegetables, seeds, nuts, grains, and vegetable oils (corn, cottonseed, safflower, sesame, soybean, and sunflower oils). Omega-3 fats are found in fish, vegetable oils, nuts (especially walnuts), flax seeds, flaxseed oil, and leafy vegetables. Fish like salmon, trout, mackerel, sardines, and herring are loaded with omega-3, as well as high quality proteins and other nutrients.

Because omega-6 competes with omega-3 in the body, excessive intake of omega-6 can inhibit omega-3 function, and therefore, a healthy diet should contain a balanced ratio of omega-6 to omega-3 (1:1, or at worst, 4:1). Unfortunately, modern Western diets have omega-6:omega-3 ratios around 15:1, meaning there is too much omega-6, and the ability of omega-3 to find its target is all but annihilated due to the fierce competition with omega-6. This imbalance is thought to be largely due to high-fat diets in which the fats come mostly from processed foods and oils. To avoid such imbalances in our own diets, we need to eat a low-fat diet with minimal processed foods and with naturally occurring omega-3 fatty acids.

Your Personal Categorization. Stop thinking of food as "good" or "bad." Instead, start to categorize food choices into anytime, sometimes, rarely, and almost never. Try to eat more "anytime" foods while limiting the "rarely" foods to monthly and the "almost never" foods to every three to six months.

Be careful about assuming the quality of a food without researching it. Many times, people have misconceptions about what is actually healthy. For example, when I was growing up, I continually overheard my grandparents talking about their new diet for the week, and it never failed that the most common breakfast items were dried toast or half of a bagel. Early in my life, I settled in my mind the idea that bagels were a "health food." Years later, during my freshman year in college, I became increasingly concerned as I flew right past the "freshman fifteen" weight gain. I decide to start inserting healthy meals into my bad eating habits. Lucky for me, or so I thought, a new bagel shop had just opened nearby. Every couple of days for the rest of the year, I entered the shop and ordered my standard—a giant bagel with extra cream cheese ("extra," because, when I was a child, my parents were always trying to get me to eat cheese, so I assumed it was good for me!). I washed it down with a bottle of blackberry-flavored water. Despite my attempt to slow my weight gain, it took off like a rocket. I stopped eating the bagels the next year, when I moved away from the bagel shop, but I never did figure out what had happened—until recently when the bagel experience touched my current thoughts. After adding up the calories and fat in one of those bagel "meals," I probably consumed about 850 calories and 42 grams of fat each morning. If I added a bag of chips (which I often rewarded myself with for eating such a "healthy" meal), then I actually consumed about 1,200 calories and 62 grams of fat in a single meal! And that was my "healthy" meal for the day—to go along with a whole pizza for dinner! Just eating that meal alone three times a week would have caused me to consume an extra 3,600 calories—enough for me to gain a whole pound of fat each week.

Don't be uninformed like I was with the bagel incident. For great information about the quality of foods and basic nutrition facts, see the *2015–2020 Dietary Guidelines for Americans,* the nation's trusted resource for evidence-based nutrition recommendations: https://www.cnpp.usda.gov/2015-2020-dietary-guidelines-americans.

AWARENESS OF HUNGER

Why are you eating? Are you hungry? Are you being proactive to counteract future hunger? (That is, are you telling yourself, *You'd better eat now, because we may not have time to eat later.*) Or are you just eating because everyone else is eating?

Let's say your answer is because of hunger. Most people would agree that eating to satisfy hunger is a valid reason to consume food. However, this idea begs another question: What are you hungry for? Are you eating because you are bored and hungry for something to do? Are you upset and hungry for pacification? And just how hungry are you, anyway?

Before we stick any kind of food in our mouths, we need to properly evaluate our hunger.

Types of Hunger. There are two basic types of hunger: homeostatic hunger and hedonic hunger.

* *Homeostatic hunger* is the physical manifestation of the body telling itself that it's time to eat. It is driven by complex chemical signaling in the body and brain. When energy stores in the body start running low, levels of a hormone named *ghrelin* (i.e., the "hunger hormone") start to rise. Signaling in the brain turns on, too. When we eat, this signaling mechanism is turned off. Some foods, like protein and fiber, are better at turning it off sooner and more completely than others, like artificial sweeteners and ultra-processed foods.

* *Hedonic hunger* is more of an emotional desire to eat that involves dwelling on food or maybe craving something. Hedonic hunger has more to do with

seeking pleasure than with actually needing energy and nutrients.

The two types of hunger are not completely distinct, but rather, they are more like a continuum, with each one being at opposite ends. A person who hasn't eaten for a long time is experiencing homeostatic hunger, whereas a person who wants dessert after just finishing a filling meal is experiencing hedonic hunger. Of the two types of hunger, hedonic hunger is generally tougher to deal with, and it is easier to prevent than overcome. The best way to fight hedonic hunger is to keep all tasty and tempting items out of your house and limit how often you eat them. As it's not always possible to isolate yourself from these foods, another approach is to fend off the hunger with a piece of fruit or some other healthy snack. Just being able to recognize hedonic hunger for what it is can helps with overcoming it, too.

Rating Hunger. Learning to rate our hunger is the best way to teach ourselves when to eat. Following is an adapted version of a hunger scale originally created by L. Ominchanski from the Center for Health Promotion and Wellness at MIT Medical in 1992.[22]

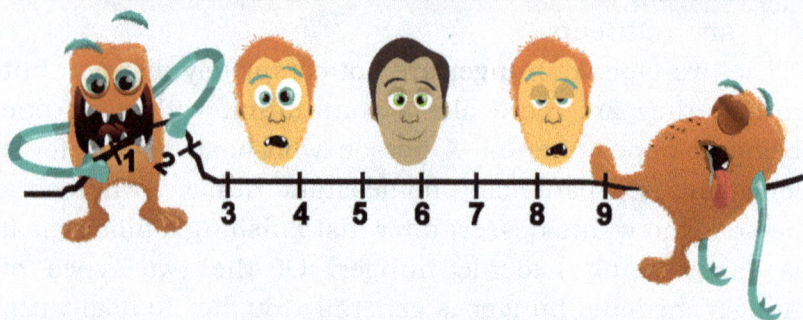

1. RAVENOUS: You may have a headache and trouble concentrating. You may feel dizzy and have trouble with coordination. You are totally depleted of energy and may want or even need to lie down.

2. HANGRY (a mix of hungry and angry): You can't seem to tolerate anything. You're irritable, cranky, and very hungry, with little energy to spare. You may even feel nauseated. You are at the stage of being famished.

3. HUNGRY: The urge to eat is strong, and you feel an emptiness in your stomach. Your coordination and concentration begin to wane.

4. HUNGER PANGS: You're starting to think about food, but the thoughts may come and go. Your body is giving you the signal that you might want to eat soon. You are a little hungry.

5. NEUTRAL: Your body has enough fuel to keep it going and is physically and psychologically just starting to feel satisfied.

6. SATISFIED: You're fully at the point of satisfaction.

7. FULL: You're past the point of satisfaction, yet you can still "find room" for a little more.

8. STUFFED: You are actually starting to hurt.

9. UNCOMFORTABLE: You feel heavy, tired, and bloated. You no longer feel like socializing; you'd rather be by yourself or go to bed.

10. PAINFULLY FULL AND/OR SICK: You are physically miserable. You don't want to move and feel like you never want to look at food again.

Make this scale part of your daily life to assess your levels of hunger.

1 or 2: Eat with caution, because it's easy to overeat when you are this hungry.

3 or 4: It's time to eat. This is when you will have the most self-control and can practice mindful eating.

7 through 10: You have eaten enough food. If you find yourself poking around in the fridge, ask yourself why and whether it could be due to boredom, stress, an unsettled emotion like grief, or an attempt to procrastinate a task needing your attention. During these stages, remind yourself that you are full and don't need to eat.

Cravings. Pickles and ice cream during pregnancy, chocolate during the menstrual cycle, etc.—everyone has had a food craving at some point in their lives. Most cravings are elicited when we catch a glimpse or a reminder of a beloved food that we haven't eaten in a while. Other cravings can be associated with emotional seasons in our lives, like when we are experiencing stress or grief. Some are even due to physical needs within our body.

In the medical and scientific community, there is a debate on whether the body can elicit cravings when it has deficiencies. Personally, I believe it can happen and I have experienced it firsthand. When I was a teenager, I had the worst eating habits ever, and I never consumed anything that had decent nutritional value. There came a time when I began to have a weird craving for vitamin C pills. Just the thought of the taste of them would make my mouth water. For many of you, this might seem like nothing, but for anyone who has tasted a vitamin C pill, you understand the significance of this craving. Vitamin C is the kind of pill that you toss to the back of your throat, trying to miss your tongue altogether—these pills are bitter beyond despair. But during this time of strange cravings, though, I would suck on that daily Vitamin C pill like it was a piece of candy. It was like heaven blossoming in my mouth at that time. Eventually, my body must have realized that my vitamin C levels were sufficient, because the flavor of the pills reverted back to "gross" to my palate, and I stopped taking them.

Other claims about nutritional-based cravings include hunger for meat due to an iron deficiency; for dirt due to a lack of B-12, folate, or iron; for chocolate due to a magnesium deficiency; and for sugary or salty junk food due to a zinc deficiency.

In some individuals, cravings may actually be related to nutritional deficiencies; however, there is a lack of proof in published scientific and medical literature, and most cases are purely anecdotal, like mine and my friend's. Most cravings are driven by a hedonic hunger for pleasure foods and are fleeting in nature; for example, someone craving pizza could satisfy the craving by eating a few slices on a single occasion. However, if the craving was based on a nutritional deficiency, the person would likely have a continual craving for foods higher in nutritional value, like red peppers, Brussels sprouts, and kale, as we previously discussed. [23] Nevertheless, some cravings are real, and anyone who continues to experience a strong and unusual food craving should discuss it with their medical doctor.

AWARENESS OF PERSONAL CONSUMPTION AND ACTIVITY

Before I started tracking my food consumption, it was nothing for me to unconsciously dip into every candy bowl available (especially ones in waiting areas), or to snatch a cookie from every passing tray. When sitting at the dinner table, I never really knew how much I ate, because as an item disappeared from my plate, I would immediately replace it. Also, before tracking my intake, I knew nearly nothing about nutrition, and I had no idea how many calories or fat grams I was consuming. Remember my bagel story? I was clueless! But on January 26, 2014, I started logging my food consumption in an app, and my food life has never been the same.

Exercise deception was another thing I had to overcome. For most of my life, I've been fairly active, but on many occasions, I overestimated my actual participation. For example, I remember having a gym membership and thinking that I went to work out all the time. However, upon closer examination, I realized that wasn't the case. In reality, I went an average of once a week, and while there, I might walk two laps while socializing and then whip out two minutes on the treadmill (because that's how long it took my heart to feel like it would jump out of my chest). I might even have done a few arm exercises with the lighter-weight dumbbell. On my "hard" days, I would have swum anywhere from twenty to forty laps. Most of the time, though, I spent a total of about ten minutes actually exercising—and none of it with any intensity. Clearly, back then I wasn't the fitness girl I thought I was. On November 5, 2015, I logged my first CrossFit experience in my app, and just as happened with my diet, my fitness life has never been the same.

The power of a food/exercise diary is indisputable in my mind. If you take only one piece of advice from this whole book, let it be this: Keep a daily diary of your eating and exercise habits!

Types of Diaries. With all the technology available, there are several options for keeping a diary. If you want an online one, then check out the food and activity tracker from the USDA: https://www.supertracker.usda.gov. Mobile apps are another convenient way to track food consumption and exercise. Following are some of the best apps for food journaling according to *Redbook* (May 2017).[24]

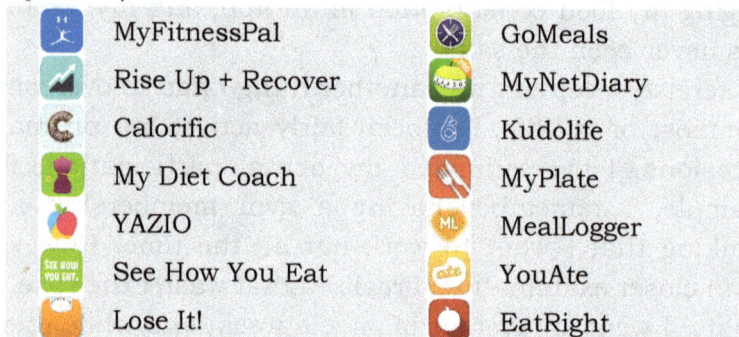

	MyFitnessPal		GoMeals
	Rise Up + Recover		MyNetDiary
	Calorific		Kudolife
	My Diet Coach		MyPlate
	YAZIO		MealLogger
	See How You Eat		YouAte
	Lose It!		EatRight

Some of these apps let the user log their exercise as well as the food they eat, whereas some are just for a person's diet. I personally use MyFitnessPal, and I have since that monumental date back in 2014.

Advantages of Apps. Following are a handful of advantages to using apps for staying aware of your personal consumption.

* *Apps Are Convenient.* These days, it's doubtful that anyone goes anywhere without a cell phone—even to the toilet! This is why apps are so handy. They are accessible at all times, and they have reminder

capabilities that can be programmed for your personal needs.

With most diary apps, you can see your progress with beautiful charts, and you can even export your data for other uses. The main reason I started logging my food and changing the way I ate was so that I could stop taking cholesterol medicine. After keeping a food diary for six months, I was able to export charts of my cholesterol and fat consumption to take with me to my annual physical examination. And when my daughter was having stomach issues, we were able to use her food diary in solving the problem.

I personally believe that one day all insurance companies will offer lower rates for people who can prove they have adopted healthier lifestyles. Some are doing it now. In my family's current personal medical coverage, we are given the option of a monthly reduction in our rates if we link our fitness tracker to our account and show that we are meeting certain minimal requirements. Also, social media platforms have observed my fitness profile activity and sent me offers for discounts from life insurance companies if I can prove my performance at a certain level on well-known high-intensity workouts (i.e., Murph). It's only a matter of time before insurance companies offer similar discounts for access to our electronic food diaries.

* *Apps Teach You to Negotiate Food Choices.* By using an app to plan your meal, you learn to negotiate your eating habits. For example, if you must choose between two competing options, after seeing the nutritional information, including that related to calorie and fat content, you can choose one or the other, or you can negotiate the amounts you eat of each, doing something

like eating half of a serving of each one (i.e., *If I eat only half of this, I can then eat more of that...*).

If you use an app like MyFitnessPal, which lets you search for foods by restaurant name and then pull up their menu offerings, you can compare all of the dishes to decide which best fits your dietary goals. One of my favorite things about using this app is that I can plan my meals for big days. For example, if I know that I'm going to go to an amazing restaurant for dinner, I can decide ahead which meal I will eat and enter it into the app earlier in the day. (And if I've never been to that restaurant before, then I can check out their online menu and decide upon a dish before I arrive.) This way, the calories and fat are already accounted for, and I can then negotiate the earlier meals of that day to meet my goals. If I were to wait and enter the meal later, unless I've planned really well, I'm stuck finding something on the restaurant menu that fits the calorie count and fat content I still have left for that day. I don't know about you, but I'd rather skimp on a routine meal than skimp on a meal for a special occasion!

* *Apps Can Offer Full-Time Accountability and Support.* An old proverb says that "stolen waters are sweet, and food obtained in secret is delicious!"[25] I can personally attest that this can be true! When I was a very young child (somewhere between three and five years old), I wasn't permitted to drink soda. I soon developed a work-around solution to my soda problem—by sneaking into the kitchen, cozying up the carton of empty sixteen-ounce glass soda bottles, and turning up each one to get any last dribbles of lingering sweetness that were in each one. Sometimes I would secretly visit the carton multiple times a day, looking for one more delicious

drop. I continued this sneaky habit until one tragic day. You see, my parents were smokers, and one thing they loved to do was to drop their cigarette butts into the empty soda bottles. On that unforgettable day, my secret habit was eradicated—with a mouth full of ashes followed by projectile vomiting!

Another advantage of using an app for your food/exercise diary is that you can connect with other people for support and accountability. In the app I use, I can let everyone on the app, or just my connected friends, see what I'm doing. No more eating in secret!

David and I lead a fitness group, and our members are encouraged to use the diary app along with us. Almost everyone accepts the suggestion to keep an electronic food diary, and it never takes long for the testimonies to come rolling in. People can't believe how much seeing what they are eating each day changes the way they think about food. Suddenly they realize self-accountability on a whole new level. In addition, they began to appreciate the accountability they now have to others in the group.

AWARENESS OF PROPER PORTION SIZES

Portion sizes started increasing in the late 1970s, rose sharply in the 1980s,[26] and have been growing ever since. Anyone who regularly eats out in restaurants has witnessed this evolution of larger serving sizes, and the ever-expanding average American waistline further testifies to this fact.

Years ago, the meal you ordered likely took up less than half the space on your plate, but now dishes arrive at the table with food spilling over, and to top it off, the plates are no longer dinner size, but look more like platters!

Why did this start? The food industry capitalized on the consumer's concern about "value" and led us to accept that larger portion sizes are a better bargain. The problem was further propagated by the industry's continual manipulation of serving sizes on their food labels in order to make their nutrition labels look the best. Exposure to larger portions, and constantly changing serving sizes on labels, have distorted our perceived consumption norms. Now folks don't have a grasp about appropriate amounts to eat. Today's food portions are often much larger than dietary guidelines recommend, and no one even recognizes this discrepancy. It's no surprise that increased serving sizes have been identified as contributing to the obesity epidemic.

What Counts as a Serving. Don't let the food industry define your food serving sizes. A better bet is to use the recommendations from the USDA. Following are some general guidelines about appropriate serving sizes of foods.

GRAINS
Bread, Cereal, Rice & Pasta

1 slice bread
~ 1 cup cereal
½ cup rice or pasta

Vegetables

1 cup raw, leafy vegetables
½ cup other vegetables
¾ cup vegetable juice

Fruit

1 medium apple,
banana, or orange
½ cup chopped fruit
¾ cup fruit juice

Milk, Yogurt & Cheese

1 cup milk or yogurt
1.5 oz natural cheese
2 oz processed cheese

2–3 oz cooked lean
meat, poultry, or fish
½ cup cooked dry
beans
1 egg = 1/3 cup nut =
1 oz lean meat
2 T peanut butter

Meat, Poultry Fish, Dry Beans, Eggs & Nuts

It's important to make sure you are properly estimating portion sizes so that you don't underestimate amounts and unintentionally sabotage your efforts of tracking your daily consumption.

To gain a sense of appropriate food amounts, measure your food using scales and cups until you can estimate with accuracy. If, while measuring, you always compare the amount to your finger or hand size (or some other visual reference), then when you are away from home and don't have access to your measuring "tools," you'll still be able to make an estimate.

Other Visual References to Use When Estimating Portion Amounts

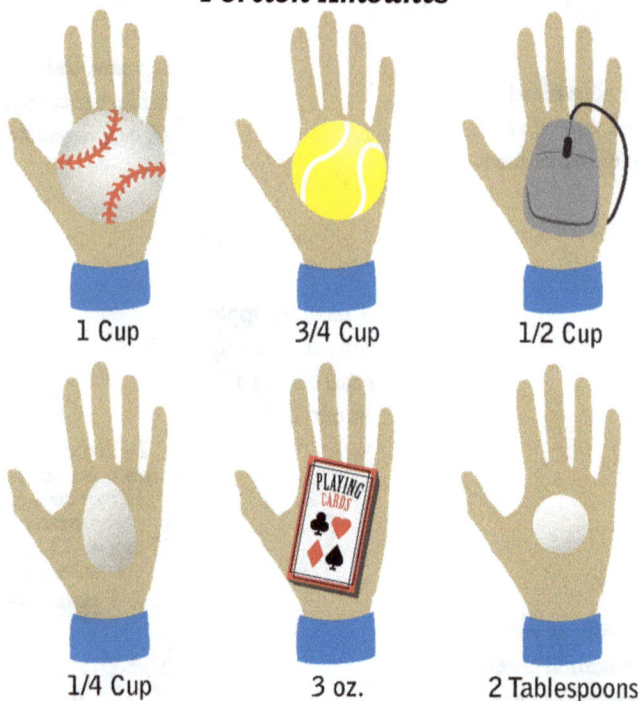

1 Cup	3/4 Cup	1/2 Cup
1/4 Cup	3 oz.	2 Tablespoons

Power of Container Size. When portion sizes increased over the years, container size was forced to expand, as well. In today's society, restaurants use larger dinner plates, and fast food comes in supersized containers. In fact, fast-food container sizes have grown so much that automobile manufacturers have actually installed larger cup holders in newer models to accommodate these new sizes.

At first thought, someone might think that overeating is due to an excessive amount of food being present and that the larger container plays no part. However, research shows that large containers have a subconscious psychological effect on consumers despite their contents. In one study, participants were served either a medium portion of chocolate candies in a small or large container, or a large portion of the candy in a large container.[27] Participants who were given candy in the larger container ate more than double than those given the same amount of candy in a smaller container. This research suggests that larger containers stimulate food intake.

In another study, moviegoers in Philadelphia were randomly given a medium or a large container of free popcorn that was either fresh or stale. Moviegoers who were given fresh popcorn ate more when it was served in large containers. This influence of container size was so powerful that even when the popcorn was perceived as tasting bad, people *still* ate more popcorn when eating from a large container than from a medium-sized one.[28]

With all the various shapes and sizes of plates and bowls (especially in restaurants), in addition to the assorted portion sizes, it can be hard to estimate how much food is actually being served to you. The next time your food order arrives, evaluate the container or plate size *independent of* the amount of food it contains, and vice versa.

Can you see the effect plate size has on portion size? It's the same amount of food on each plate, but the consumer would likely feel cheated (and maybe left feeling psychologically hungry) if they were served the plates on the right.

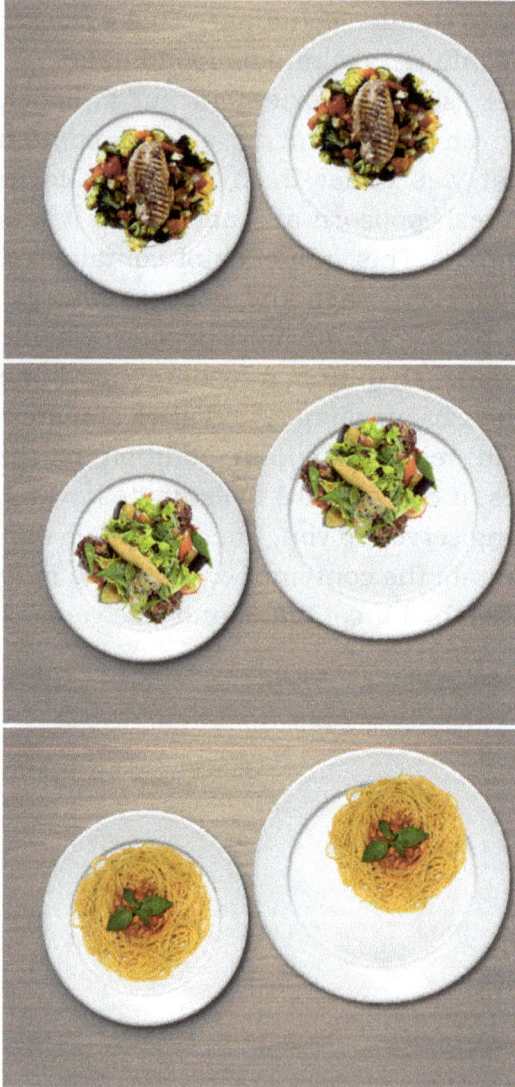

Dual-Column Nutrition Labels. One way to battle this growing serving size problem is the idea of dual-column nutrition labels. Currently, most nutrition labels show a single column that lists the amount of nutrients per serving of the food (keep in mind that the entire package may contain multiple servings). With a dual-column label, beside this serving size column would be another column listing the amount of nutrients consumed if the person were to consume the entire package of food. Because most consumers are not interested in doing mental math while deciding how much to eat of something, by having both columns (one to show information for each *serving* consumed, and the other to show information for each *package* consumed), the consumer might be less likely to overeat. Research shows that dual-column nutrition labels can decrease snack-food consumption.[29]

Dual Nutrition Label

Nutrition Facts

About 2.5 servings per container
Serving size   About 11 chips (28g)

	Per serving		Per package	
Calories	**150**		**400**	
		% DV*		% DV*
Total Fat	9g	12%	25g	32%
Saturated Fat	1.5g	7%	3.5g	18%
Trans Fat	0g		0g	
Cholesterol	0mg	0%	0mg	0%
Sodium	160mg	7%	430mg	19%
Total Carb.	16g	6%	41g	15%
Dietary Fiber	1g	5%	3g	12%
Total Sugars	1g		3g	
Incl. Added Sugars	<1g	1%	1g	3%
Protein	2g		5g	
Vitamin D	0mcg	0%	0mcg	0%
Calcium	10mg	0%	30mg	2%
Iron	0.5mg	2%	1.4mg	6%
Potassium	340mg	6%	890mg	15%
Vitamin C		6%		15%

The % Daily Value (DV) tells you how much a nutrient in a serving of food contributes to a daily diet. 2,000 calories a day is used for general nutrition advice.

Visualize the Actual Size of Your Stomach. The stomach is the most variable organ in the body in terms of size. Generally, about twelve inches by six inches, it has a capacity of about one liter in an average adult when empty, but it can be distended to hold up to four liters (more than one gallon).[30] I personally think of my own stomach as being about the same size as two of my fists.

One way to estimate an appropriate amount to eat is to compare the food on your plate to your stomach size. Visualize the amount of food sitting before you all clumped together in a ball. How big is that ball? This is a rough estimate of how much your stomach will be distended after eating all of it. Now imagine the actual amount that you would be comfortable having inside of your body.

Think about caloric density when you are deciding what to eat. For example, if a small amount of the food has a large number of calories, then it is considered to have a high caloric density. Try to choose foods that are lower in caloric density or that will bring you satiation easier. Imagine that someone had the option of eating 400 calories and their choices were oil, beef, or vegetables (see the picture below). Which choice will make the person feel more satisfied and full? The vegetables will, because they have a lower caloric density.

Caloric Density

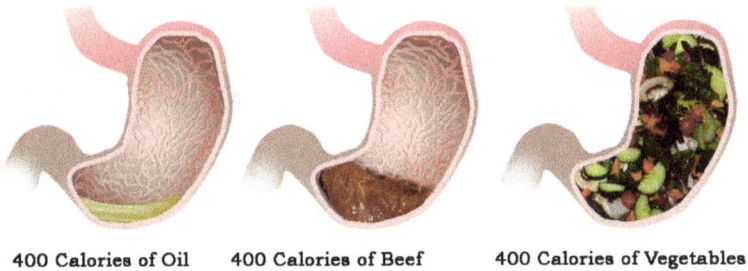

| 400 Calories of Oil | 400 Calories of Beef | 400 Calories of Vegetables |

Stretch receptors are located throughout the stomach. When they are triggered by food, they send signals to your brain to tell you to stop eating. With high fiber, whole plant foods, you can eat the most quantity for the least amount of calories.

(c) 2012 Julieanna Hever, MS, RD, CPT www.PlantBasedDietitian.com
Illustration by Sherri Nestorowich www.sherrinest.wix.com/art
Graphic used with permission.

Understanding Weight versus Volume. When assessing portion sizes, it is important to understand the differences in weight versus volume, especially when using a food journal, because you can be measuring one way and seeing proof in your journal that you're eating right, but then you might not be losing weight. The reason is that you may not actually be eating the portion sizes you think you are.

In general, *weight* is for measuring dry foods, and *volume* is to measure liquid foods. However, serving sizes on packaging will likely include both.

Errors can arise when you use volume as a way to measure dry food, because one method may underrepresent the actual amount. Another problem with measuring dry food by volume is that the size of the food bits can affect its volume. For example, consider my favorite cereal, which has a serving size of one cup (29 grams) and is 110 calories. But what if my cereal box was mishandled and all the cereal was crushed into crumbs? Now when I eat one cup, I am consuming about 25 percent more calories than I thought I was.

Intact   **Crushed**

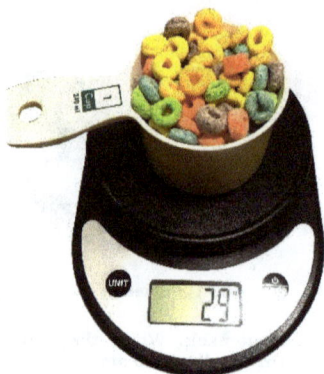 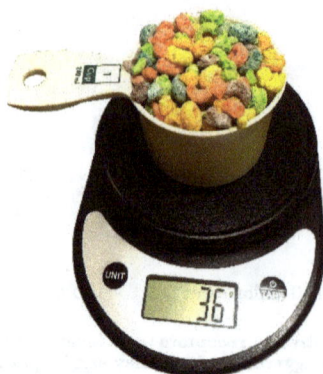

You might think that a twenty-seven-calorie difference is not that much, but over time, these seemingly small differences add up. If I experienced this margin of error consistently with most of my foods, I could unknowingly end up consuming almost 1,900 calories in a day when my target was only 1,500.

The take-home message for learning to estimate portion sizes is to measure your food by the proper means, even if only for a little while, to better understand what actual serving sizes should be.

Taming Your Monster Appetite by Jennifer Minigh

Don't Invite It into the House

The biggest struggle with temptation isn't in our home— it's in the grocery stores and the restaurants. If you don't buy junk food and keep it in your house, then you won't have to struggle with not eating it. Prevention is 99 percent of the cure.

DON'T FALL PREY TO INTENTIONAL MARKETING

Research shows that four key product cues affect whether we will like something: 1) its perceived satiety, which is the feeling of fullness or satisfaction after eating, 2) its brand and labeling, 3) its price, and 4) its emotional impact on decision-making.[31] Marketing experts are capitalizing on these findings and are creating ploys to stimulate buyers to make purchases. It is important for us to recognize these "temptation cues" so that we can mitigate their effect on our choices. Knowledge is powerful, and when we recognize these marketing tactics, we will stop falling prey to them.

Using Our Senses Against Us. Food is one of the few things in life that can be enjoyed by all five of our senses, and marketers look for ways to engage all five to entice us. Lord, help us all if "smell-o-vision" ever comes to pass! Who could withstand the smell of freshly baked bread, warm cookies, or frying bacon?

A study led by marketing professors at Brigham Young University and the University of Washington showed that certain sensory descriptions can affect whether someone will immediately purchase something or postpone it to another time.[32] In one experiment, subjects read one of two reviews for a fictional restaurant. One review described the taste and touch aspects (senses that must be experienced in close proximity to our bodies), while the other emphasized sounds and sights (senses that can be experienced at a farther distance away from our bodies). After reading their assigned reviews, participants were instructed to make a reservation for the restaurant. Those who read the review focusing on the more proximal senses (i.e., taste and touch) were more likely to make a reservation closer to the present time frame.

Other scientific research has shown that when participants described foods with words that simulated eating, taste, or enjoyment, they also reported a desire to eat those foods.[33] I've witnessed this effect firsthand in the grocery store every time I go down the cereal aisle and see a box with "*snap, crackle,* and *pop*" written on it and want a fresh bowl of it!

Did you know that the actual physical pronunciation of certain words can create a desire to eat, too? When we pronounce words, the articulation of the consonants can wander around in our mouth. For example, when you say the fake word *PASOKI*, the *P* sound starts on the lips, and is followed by the *S* sound on the tongue and then the *K* sound in the back of the mouth. Pronunciation of this word creates an inward flow from the lips to the throat and simulates eating. In contrast, if you were to pronounce the fake word *KASOPI*, the movement is the reverse, and it simulates an expectorant-like action, or regurgitation. In one study, researchers investigated whether the pronunciation of a word assigned for a particular food would affect a person's desire to consume it.[34] Various dishes and food items were labeled with names whose consonants either wandered from front to back in the mouth (like *PASOKI*) or from back to front (like *KASOPI*). Those items that bore an inwardly wandering name were rated higher in tastiness than those with an outward one.

Rest assured that all of this research does not go unnoticed by marketing people in the food industry. They look for ways to make foods more desirable, thereby increasing sales and profits. Can you imagine how valuable a list of words that induce salivation or stimulate the desire to eat would be to these folks?

The next time you see the packaging of an unhealthy food and it makes you want to immediately tear into it, take a moment to notice any marketing ploys that could be appealing to your senses.

Using Triggers and Cues. Have you ever experienced the ringing of a dinner bell at a buffet when fresh rolls were put out? Have you ever heard the approaching chime of an ice cream truck? Or have you ever seen the "Hot Now" sign burning brightly at the doughnut shop in your neighborhood?? (I don't know about you, but just thinking about that glowing sign...oh, goodness...my mouth waters like Pavlov's dogs!) These are marketing triggers.

* *Branding Symbols.* The recognition of a symbol as an international brand is a dream of any company. Imagine how many folks across the world recognize the Golden Arches, which represent the most famous fast-food restaurant in history. Or how many people could tell you the manufacturer's name of the electronic device that has the logo of a bitten apple on it?

  Oftentimes, logos may have subliminal messages that may not be readily apparent, but with increased exposure, will eventually influence the consumer's choices.

The Wendy's logo promotes a personal and "home-cooked" feeling. A closer look at Wendy's collar will reveal the word "mom."

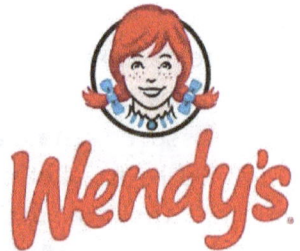

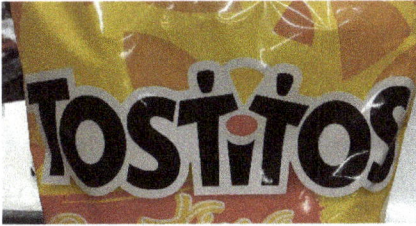

Notice that the two *T*s of the logo are people dipping a tortilla chip into a bowl of salsa on top of the letter *i*.

McDonald's golden arches are actually French fries.

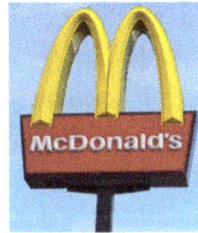

Often when folks are in a hurry, but they still need to eat, they may opt for fast food; therefore, these types of restaurants have become synonymous with speed and convenience. In fact, the power of these symbols surpasses the eating domain. In one study, even an unconscious exposure to fast-food symbols increased participants' reading speed when they were under no time pressure.[35] In addition, thinking about fast food increased their preferences for time-saving products despite other products available for consideration. More strikingly, though, exposure to fast-food symbols reduced the participants' willingness to save and made them prefer immediate but smaller gains over greater future returns, even if it meant economic harm.

* *Colors*. We wouldn't normally eat a turquoise hamburger or black sour cream. Instead, we prefer that the color of food matches its flavor, and the food industry meets our expectations by using various food dyes.

About 70 percent of a typical American's diet is from processed foods. [36] The act of processing a food substance can change its color, and most of the time, the resulting color is not that appetizing. As such, nearly all processed foods contain added dyes to make them appear more palatable. Edible spray paint is also available and can be applied to any food.

Food coloring is like cosmetics for your food. Without food dye, hot dogs would be gray. Sounds yummy, right? Eating is a full sensory experience, and the sight of your food is just as important as its taste when it comes to enjoyment. Ask yourself whether that raspberry slushy would taste the same if you couldn't see that vivid color climbing up the straw, or even worse, if you didn't have a blue mouth afterward.

The food industry capitalizes on our emotional connection with color. They carefully decide the final color of their food products, as well as the packaging in which they present it to us. The food industry keeps this type of thinking in mind when it comes to advertising to consumers. For example, the color red is associated with passion, hurriedness, and the "red effect," which is the influence of the color red on our decision-making processes that causes us to prefer things in red.[37] Orange and yellow have the potential to induce hunger. It's no surprise, then, to see fast-food restaurants decorated with these three colors. Other colors are used as triggers for other responses. Green and earth tones induce sentiments of something being eco-friendly, natural, organic, and healthy. White implies purity, cleanliness, and wholeness. Black is often unappetizing, and blue can inhibit hunger; therefore, these colors are used judiciously in food packaging. In fact, the color blue is often used in weight-loss programs. Children prefer foods that are red, green, orange, or yellow—in that order.[38]

In one study,[39] scientists explored the effect of food packaging color on the perceived healthfulness of the food product. The results showed that yellow, blue, green, and red were found to be suggestive of health, while heather, pink, and green suggested an artificial, and thus unhealthy product.

In another study,[40] participants judged whether pairs of colorful sugar-coated, chocolate candies (similar to M&Ms) had the same flavors. These candies came in eight different colors, but only two different flavors. Orange candies that had been manufactured for the UK market contained orange-flavored chocolate, whereas all of the other colors contained milk chocolate. The candies manufactured for other markets all contained milk chocolate, no matter the candy color. By using these candies from different markets, the researchers were able to present pairs of candy that differed in color but not flavor, flavor but not color, and both color and flavor. The results demonstrated that people's expectations concerning color-flavor associations can modify their flavor discrimination responses, even for a familiar food product such as candy.

Pay attention to the packaging of foods and look past the color to see the true nutritional value and quality of the food. You can also use color to your advantage in restaurants. My family likes to eat at a popular buffet that has various colored plates to choose from. Try using the blue plates, and avoid the red, yellow, or orange ones. You may find that the color affects what you invite onto your plate.

*   *Spokespeople/Endorsers.* For the purposes of this book, a spokesperson/endorser is a well-known person who uses his or her fame to help promote a product or a service. Generally, these are people whom the consumer is expected to either identify with or admire, and they are often celebrities, superheroes, or cartoon characters.

One of the pioneers of celebrity endorsements in terms of food marketing and packaging was General Mills, with their Wheaties cereal boxes. In 1934, they began putting famous athletes on their box covers (the first of whom was Lou Gehrig). My personal favorite was manufactured in 1984, when sixteen-year-old Mary Lou Retton became the first American woman to win an Olympic medal of any kind in gymnastics and she was pictured on the box. Just like everyone else who sees their favorite hero on the cover, I wanted to eat Wheaties so I could be as strong and graceful as Mary Lou was.

Children and their parents are probably the biggest target for spokesperson marketing tactics, and research proves how susceptible they are. In studies with children, taste ratings for foods were highest for products that included spokes-characters on the packaging.[41,42]

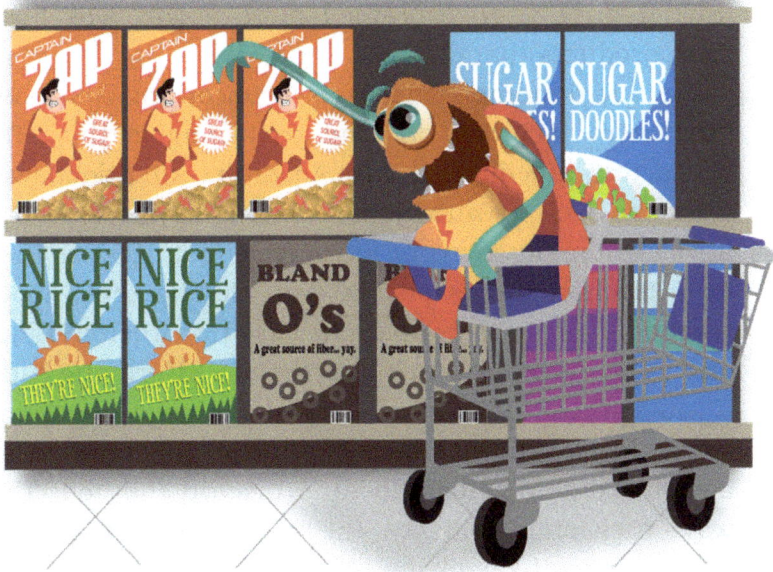

Another study tested whether the presence of both child-targeted and parent-targeted (i.e., nutrition-focused) marketing cues on food packaging was associated with the nutritional content of the products.[43] The analysis was performed on foods from a supermarket in southeastern United States and was comprised of 403 food packages chosen randomly from the supermarket's online portal, along with all 312 products from the cereal aisle. Results showed that the presence of parent-directed nutritional cues was linked to more nutritious content (e.g., less sugar, less saturated fat, more fiber) while the presence of child-targeted cues was associated with less nutritious content. The researchers concluded that products designed to engage children with their packaging are significantly less nutritious than foods that do not. Furthermore, products that try to engage both child and parent consumers were significantly less healthy in crucial ways (e.g., contained more sugar, less fiber) than products that did not.

The take-home message concerning spokes-characters included on food packaging is this: The characters are likely a ruse to divert attention away from the lack of nutritional content in the food. My advice? Stop buying your kids cereal just because their favorite character is on the box. Buying these foods teaches kids to buy products based on their feelings and to be susceptible to inappropriate advertising cues. If you can't avoid buying the cereal, then another option would be to bring it home and place the cereal in an airtight container for use—and discard the box. This way, they child will see the container and not the character on the package.

In terms of endorsers in general, it is always important to keep in mind that spokespeople are paid money or given some sort of compensation to say that they like the product. Sometimes it's human nature to forget this fact.

* *Nutritional Cues.* Nutrition-related marketing buzzwords such as *gluten-free, organic, natural, whole grain,* and *antioxidant* are hot trends in today's food industry. Most nutritional cues, however, don't really mean anything, and many of them are there to divert attention away from real problems, such as high amounts of saturated fat, sodium, or sugar. [44] In addition, these cues are used more often on products marketed toward children than products marketed toward adults. Following are some standard buzzwords that may not mean what you think they do.

"Organic" does not mean the same thing as "certified organic." For a product to be "certified organic," it must meet specific standards set forth by the USDA.

"Cage free" means that the birds were raised without cages, but it does not mean they weren't raised in overcrowded indoor spaces at large factory farms.

"Free range" labels can be used if the animal had any access to the outdoors each day, but it does not ensure that the animal ever actually was able to roam freely. Also, the outdoor area could be fenced.

"Natural" meat and poultry products, according to the USDA, cannot contain artificial colors, artificial flavors, preservatives, or other artificial ingredients, and they should be "minimally processed." However, this label says nothing about how the animals were raised, what they were fed, or whether antibiotics or hormones were used. Some experts believe that the USDA should regulate the "all natural" food cue, because this claim is likely to mislead most consumers.[45]

"Pasture-raised" or "pastured" means that animals spent some unspecified time outdoors on pasture, feeding on grass or forage.

The coloring of food packaging can give false nutrition cues, too. For example, people are more likely to assume that foods with green labels are more nutritious, and food marketing experts exploit this assumption.

* *Fitness Cues.* Some manufactures attempt to entice people who are trying to eat healthy by including fitness cues on food packaging. Examples of these cues include images of people exercising or playing a sport, or words like *active, fitness,* or *fuel.*

Research shows that consumers feel less guilty and consider themselves closer to their desired fitness levels after having consumed food that comes packaged with fitness cues.[46] In general, fitness branding tends to promote eating more and exercising less; it undermines fitness goals and hinders efforts to lose or maintain weight. Don't be fooled! Fitness-labeled foods are not a replacement for physical activity, and they can actually undo much of your hard work.

Most people wouldn't think twice before eating a "healthy" energy bar, but they would balk at eating a candy bar. Can you honestly see much difference between the two examples below? Before you consume any sort of "health food," make sure you read the label first to make sure you know exactly what you're getting.

a popular energy bar	**a popular candy bar**
made with "smooth, organic peanut butter mixed with crunchy peanut pieces"	(and my personal favorite) "packed with roasted peanuts, nougat, caramel, and milk chocolate"
• 40 grams of carbs	• 33 grams of carbs
• 11 grams of protein	• 4 grams of protein
• 7 grams of fat	• 12 grams of fat
• 260 calories	• 250 calories

Portion Size Manipulation. Unit size and serving size are not always the same. Unit size is the number of units in which a given amount of food is divided. Serving size (or portion size) is the amount of a food or drink that is typically served. Consider a bag of cookies that includes twenty cookies. While the unit size is one cookie (and there are twenty units in the bag), the serving size can be either a whole bag of twenty cookies or some smaller number of cookies.

Food companies get to define their own unit and serving sizes of their products, and many times they are not consistent, even within a particular product. For example, last week, David purchased beef jerky on two different occasions. Both times, he chose the same brand and flavor; the only difference was that one of the packages had more than double the amount of jerky than the other. (I'm sure that many of you have also opted for the larger quantities of items to get a lower price. It's the bulk-buying mentality that wholesale club stores have successfully programmed into our minds.) When David started to compare the nutrition labels of the two, he noticed that each one cited a different serving size. For the smaller package, the serving size was 1 ounce, while for the larger package it was 3 ounces.

To most consumers, differences in serving sizes of products go unnoticed, and the food industry is counting on this. Why? Because they can manipulate the sizes in order to make the nutritional information of the food more appealing and to be able to make certain nutritional claims. Here's a story to illustrate the power of serving size deception.

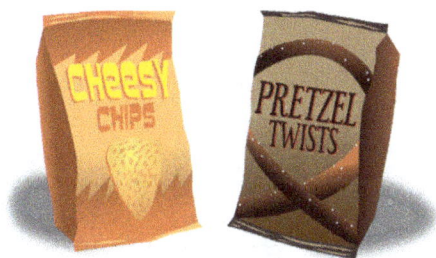

John is on a long road trip to the beach and stops at the next gas station for a quick snack to hold him over before reaching the hotel. He decides on a small bag of chips and a soda. Although it's one small bag of chips, he wants to do the right thing and so he goes for the healthiest one. He takes a quick glance at a couple of labels to compare the calorie amounts.

Hmmm... 140 calories for a bag of Cheesy Chips—not bad! And it's lower than the other option, Pretzel Twists, which has 150 calories. John opts for the lower-calorie Cheesy Chips, pays the bill, and gets back behind the wheel, while scarfing down the whole bag and soda.

Later, when John goes to enter his snack into his food diary app, he gets a huge shock. He didn't eat 140 calories of chips. Nope. He ate 420 calories! Three times his assumed amount! How could this have happened? He thought it was only a small bag of chips...

When John was looking at the Cheesy Chips label in the store, he didn't look at the *entire* label. If he had, he would have seen that this small, snack-sized bag contained *three* servings of chips, with each serving containing 140 calories; therefore, he ate three times more than he thought he did.

Nutrition Facts		
Serving Size 1 oz (28g/About 11 chips)		
Servings Per Container About 3		
Amount Per Serving		
Calories 140	Calories from Fat 70	
		% Daily Value*
Total Fat 8g		12%
Saturated Fat 1g		6%
Trans Fat 0g		
Cholesterol 0mg		0%
Sodium 210mg		9%
Total Carbohydrate 16g		5%

Food companies bank on consumers making the same assumptions as John did, so they change their serving sizes to look better than their competitors'. In John's case, he was comparing two bags of chips that appeared to be the same size. In the bag he chose, each serving size of Cheesy Chips was 11 chips. *Only 11 chips!* Had he looked more closely at the other bag, of Pretzel Twists, he might have noticed that even though each serving of Pretzel Twists was 150 calories, he could have eaten 50 twists for each serving of it.

If you do a little math, you will see that Cheesy Chips is about 13 calories per single chip (i.e., 140 calories divided by 11 chips) while Pretzel Twists are 3 calories per single twist (i.e., 150 calories divided by 50 twists). Had the company of Cheesy Chips made each serving size to be just one more chip (12 chips instead of 11 chips), each serving of the Cheesy Chips would have been 156 calories (i.e., 13 calories per chip times 12 chips) instead of 140 calories, and it would have appeared to John more than then Pretzel Twists. When consumers would have compared the two snacks, they would have seen that Pretzel Twists contained fewer calories (150 calories) than Cheesy Chips (156 calories), and the sale may have gone to the Pretzel Twists instead.

Another reason the food industry manipulates serving sizes is to be able to place special words on the food packaging. For example, to get the words "zero trans-fat" onto a food label, the food must contain 0.5 grams or less of trans fatty acids per serving as mandated by the FDA.[47] Companies can exploit this loophole by decreasing the serving size enough to make the amount of trans fatty acids meet the requirement. Imagine a bag of miniature cookies that is labeled with "zero trans-fat." Sounds good, right? But what if the serving size was only one cookie and each cookie contained 0.5 grams of trans fatty acids? Because the cookies are less than bite size, the average person would likely eat a handful, which would be about a dozen cookies, meaning that the person would eat 6 grams of trans fatty acids instead of zero grams like the package claimed. Tricky, tricky!

LEAVE IT AT THE STORE

Where and how we shop affects what we buy. If we learn what our tendencies are, then we can better limit what we carry out of the store and into our homes.

Watch Where You Shop. When it comes to shopping, there are no shortages in types of stores. So, what determines the specific stores we choose? Most of the time, it comes down to convenience, and it is likely driven by distance to and from the store as well as access to transportation. Sometimes a convenience store is all that's accessible, or perhaps an individual must limit the number of shopping bags because he or she is using public transportation.

Research shows that shopping at convenience stores is associated with increased consumption of chips, candy, and pastries. [48] In fact, each additional trip to a convenience store increases the consumption by 3 percent. In contrast, shopping at full-service grocery stores and farmers markets is positively associated with the consumption of fresh produce. Not only do food items in convenience stores put a hurt on your wallet, they put one on your waistline, as well. If at all possible, avoid convenience stores for your grocery shopping. Opt for specialty stores instead and make weekly trips to a farmer's market. Additional research showed that participants who shopped frequently at food co-ops and specialty shops had better diet quality, lower BMI, and smaller waist size than those who did not. [49]

Watch out for surplus and bulk stores. When we buy food in bulk, we may be tempted to eat more before its freshness expires or because we feel like we need to get our money's worth. If you do buy in bulk, portion the food out into manageable meal-size quantities and store each separately until it is time to use it. Again, use the bulking approach to help your wallet and not hurt your waistline.

Watch How You Shop. Most of the time when I'm shopping it's because I've run out of everything, and I'm trying to fit a mad spree into my already-busy day. I'm usually in between meals, distracted to no end, short on patience, and consumed with my loathing of this now-urgent, procrastinated task. (Can you tell I hate shopping?) It never fails, though—the quality of my attitude and my disposition during a shopping trip mirrors the quality of food that follows me home. Following are some tools I use to help me be a better shopper and leave the bad stuff at the store.

I aim to shop with confidence. I've been known to listen to music through headphones while shopping. I chose songs that make me feel strong and confident. If I feel good about myself, then it's easier to turn down stuff that would destroy that self-image.

I aim to never shop on an empty stomach. If I shop under the influence of hunger, I'll buy everything my hands can reach, and if I can't reach it, I may use a box of spaghetti noodles to knock it off the top shelf! Also, I am more susceptible to impulse buys and advertising ploys. I end up coming home with lots of bad food, no money, and a hot pizza because I couldn't wait to get home and cook something after spending so much time eyeballing all that food.

I often chew a strong-flavored gum while I shop. It keeps me from imagining all the flavors of the chips and candies. The stronger the gum, the more powerful the inhibition. Research shows there may be another reason to chew gum while walking through a store. In one study,[50] participants rinsed their mouth with either water, a placebo, or a sweet solution while walking on a treadmill. Meanwhile, researchers collected appetite ratings from the participants and measured their energy expenditure. Participants who rinsed with the sweet solution reported lower appetite and had greater energy expenditure compared with those who rinsed with water. Is it a stretch to say that chewing a sweet-flavored gum while walking through a store will help to mitigate our appetite? Either way, it's worth a try!

I use a shopping list or a plan. I used to keep a master shopping list of all the items my family consumed and would print it out when it came time to shop. Now with the advances of technology, I use an app to keep my master list. Several chain grocery stores now have apps. My local grocery store has an app that I can use to build a master list of my personal selections. When I'm making a shopping list of my current needs, I just click on the item from my personal catalog. These apps are great, because they often include information on current sales and they offer extra coupons. Some of them even tell you which aisle the items are on. When shopping, I stick to my plan as best I can, and only divert from my list if I just forgot to add the item in the first place.

Sometimes I use online ordering or a personal shopper. Online ordering is becoming widely prevalent and wildly popular. Some stores will allow you to order and pay online. Then they gather your items and have the order ready for your drive-by pickup at your scheduled time. It's easier to avoid extra purchases when you never step a foot into the store. Another option is to hire a personal shopper. If professional shoppers are not available in your area, then consider contributing to the college fund of a local teenager. I've used the online shopping with drive-by pickup and I love it. As far as a personal shopper goes, my teenage daughter has fulfilled this need on several occasions.

I avoid the "bad aisles" like the plague. The only time I enter the "seasonal" aisle is when I need to get candy for trick-or-treaters or candy canes for my Christmas tree. On the occasions when I *must* see what's there, I just stand at the end of the aisle and scan it with my eyes without walking down it. Sometimes I feel like Moses looking over the Promised Land.

Before I start shopping, I remind myself of all the marketing ploys designed to destroy my goodwill effort. I turn on my thinking cap and turn up the suspicion knob. For more information on the pitfalls I'm referring to, see the section on *Don't Fall Prey to Intentional Marketing.*

The next time you embark on the chaotic world of grocery shopping, try some of these tactics for yourself to keep from bringing bad food home with you.

LEAVE IT AT THE RESTAURANT

Because up to a third of all the energy we get from food is consumed from restaurants,[51] leftovers become a sneaky way an appetite monster can creep into your home.

The easiest way to decrease the amount of leftovers you bring home is to order smaller portion sizes from the get-go. Many restaurants will allow customers to order lunch-sized portions instead of dinner sizes regardless of what time it is. Another option is to share a meal with someone.

If you do have unintentional leftovers, *and* the meal was healthy, then consider bringing the leftovers home with you for another healthy meal the next day. However, if the meal was a splurge meal, then enjoy it for what it was, and leave the leftovers at the restaurant.

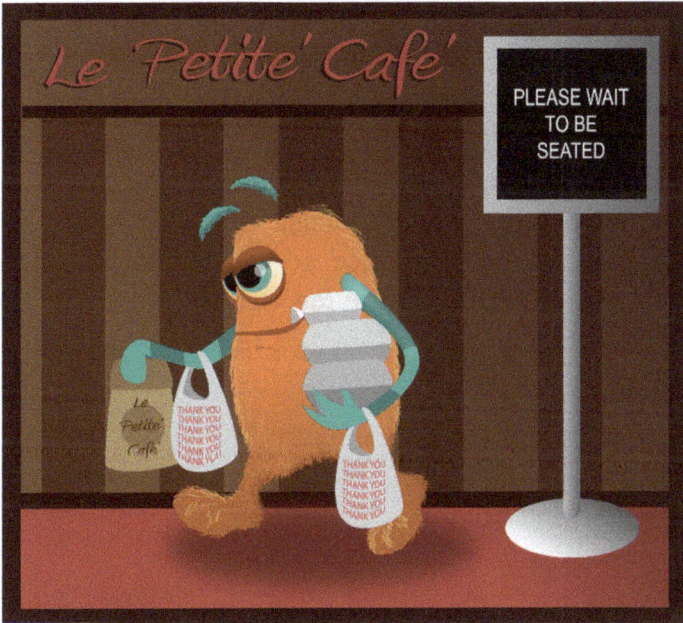

Ice cream cake. It's a favorite in our family, and it was the only type of cake my husband would consider for his fortieth birthday. While we were all enjoying a piece of the chocolatey goodness and were engaged in equally great family conversation, my husband casually asked if anyone wanted another piece. Well, of course, we didn't, because we were still finishing off the slices we had! We all continued to chat despite the ensuing cacophony coming from the kitchen sink. When we finally turned around to see what all the fuss was about, we were shocked to see the last morsel of the barely eaten, extra-large cake going down the garbage disposal. Along with it went all my dreams of second, third, fourth, and fifth helpings...that would go on for days. I mean—why else would we buy such a large cake, right? As devastated as I was, though, I wasn't surprised. In general, we don't bring home unhealthy leftovers, and we certainly don't put sweets in the freezer for later.

You may be questioning my recommendation of abandoning leftovers, and I understand. Please note that I'm not advocating wastefulness. Just ask yourself: You already paid for the meal once, so why pay for it again with weight gain and guilt? Is the few dollars' worth of leftover food worth that price?

LEAVE IT ON THE AIRWAYS

The next time you sit down to watch your favorite TV show, I dare you to count all the food cues in the program itself, and in the commercials associated with it. You'll be amazed at how much food is being pushed onto viewers. The food industry reserves no mercy for children, either. Researchers evaluated the presence of food and beverage cues in children-specific programs and found that sweet snacks were the most frequent food cue (13.3 percent), followed by sweets/candy (11.4 percent).[52]

Research shows that food cues on TV stimulates eating and snacking. In fact, one researcher noted, *"Food cues, such as the sight of appetizing food, can evoke a desire to eat, even in the absence of hunger."*[53]

Shows specifically designed about food and cooking are more popular now than ever.[54,55,56,57] It should not be surprising that frequent watching of cooking shows is associated with a higher BMI.[58] Studies have shown that watching food-related TV programs can increase people's food intake—even during the viewing.[59] It also leads to an increased consumption of calories in foods they cook for themselves afterward.[60]

Cooking shows glamorize food without regard to nutritional quality or the consequences of excess consumption, and they especially give rise to the "food porn" industry. According to Wikipedia,[61] *food porn* is:

> *a glamourized spectacular visual presentation of cooking or eating in advertisements, infomercials, blogs, cooking shows, or other visual media, foods boasting a high fat and calorie content, exotic dishes that arouse a desire to eat, or*

the glorification of food as a substitute for sex.

Just like in the "other" pornography industry, airbrushing and image sharing are common in food porn, too. Social media and photo embellishing apps fuel people's current obsession to post sensational images of their meals. [62] Professional photographers for food advertisements take it a step further and use things like shoe polish to add a nice golden-brown appearance to items like bread. Many of the images of food may not even be of real food. For example, the luscious milk you see in the cereal ad may actually be glue.

Food porn is a growing problem and is constantly coming into your home across the airways. If you are caught up in its enchantment and your health is taking a hit, then flip the switch, change the channel, or close the app. Do whatever it takes to keep it out of your home. Leave it on the airways.

Divide & Conquer

To overcome our appetites, sometimes we must use brute force to deal with the monster. The best strategy is to divide and conquer, taking it one battle at time.

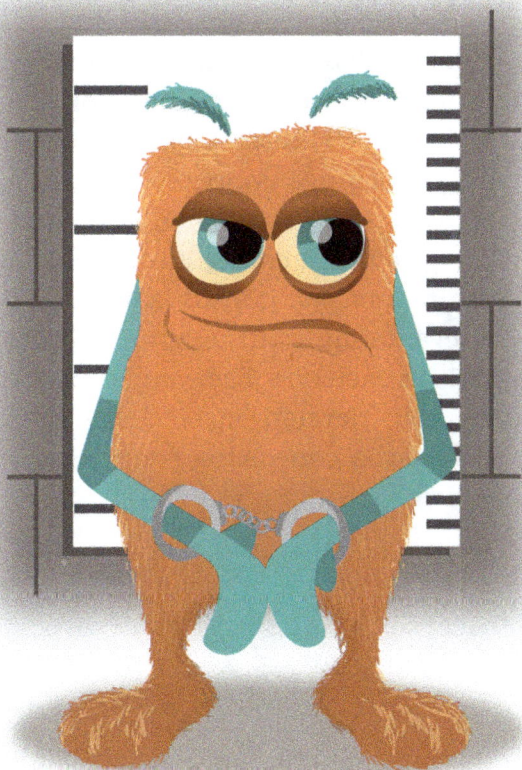

BE AWARE OF ENVIRONMENTAL EFFECTS

A very wise man once told me that we eat with our eyes first, and I totally agree. The more delicious foods look to me, the more I'm likely to eat.

Research shows that our eating environment, such as portion size, plate size, proximity to food, variety of food, and presence of distractions, can affect our consumption. In one study performed via telephone interviews asking participants about their evening meal, researchers witnessed that participants consumed more when there was an absence of salads/vegetables and when there was a wide variety of foods available.[63] Music affects our eating too; however, it may be a positive or negative influence, as studies show conflicting evidence, probably owing to people's different *taste* in music. (Pun intended.)

Understanding how our eating environment affects our personal consumption is key to gaining better eating habits. Start evaluating your eating environments and your eating style in each one. Knowing what your bad ones are will help you develop strategies that you could implement to assist in controlling your eating and reduce over consumption.

USE PROPER PORTION SIZES

Every day, we see how increased portion sizes are contributing to the rising rates of obesity. Research shows that people consume more when offered a larger portion than when offered a smaller portion, and they also eat more when their eating companion eats more. [64] In addition, increasing the portion size leads to a faster eating rate and thus a potential for overeating.[65]

For what is proper portion size, see the section about *Awareness of Personal Consumption and Activity* on page 59. Following are some ways to control portion sizes.

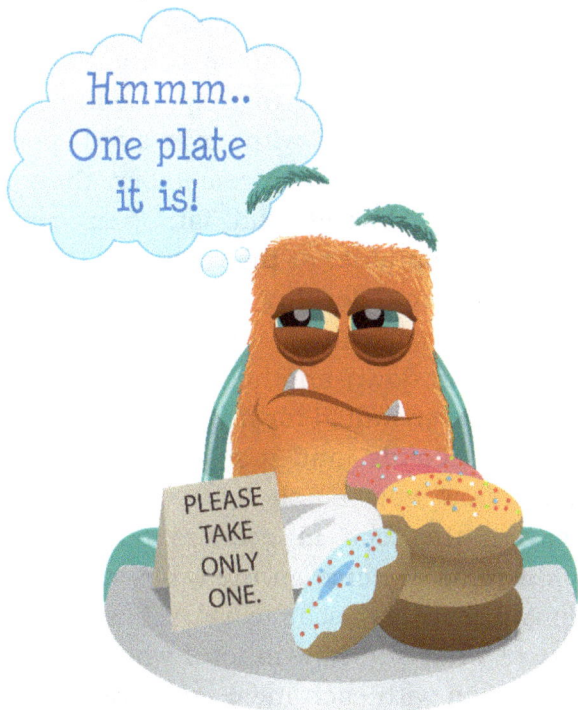

Use Smaller Plates and Bowls. In one study, participants were randomly assigned to either a group serving pasta from a large bowl (6.9-liter) or a medium bowl

(3.8-liter).[66] When the large bowl was used, participants served seventy-seven percent more pasta.

Portion Out Your Own Food. When consuming individually packaged foods, don't be tricked by single units that actually contain up to three servings each. Single items suggest portion size, but may actually be multiple servings (i.e., a small bag of chips or a candy bar). When served over-sized portions in a restaurant, immediately cut the amount on the plate in half. Move one half to one side of the plate and move the other to the other side or better yet, go ahead and put it into a to-go box. One study showed that when a take-out container was given at the start of a meal, participants consumed less, and the researchers suggested that a to-go container may be an effective environmental cue to help consumers control serving size when faced with over-sized portions at restaurants.[67] It's important to remember, though—if the meal was high in calories and fat, then conveniently "forget" the to-go container at the restaurant.

Don't Sit Near the Serving Bowls. Long ago, during typical meals at home, as an item disappeared from my plate, I would slop down another spoonful of it from the serving bowl. I never waited for my plate to be clear before going back for seconds, and just refilled as I went, so I never really knew how much I ate. At some point, we started leaving the food in cookers on the stove and countertop instead of items on the table, which forced me to consciously leave my seat to get refills and made me more aware of what and how much I was eating. Now, we use this approach with each meal, and I've also instituted it during my workday, by not keeping snacks around my desk.

Making food harder to get decreases mindless eating, and turns out, that science has shown this. Researchers asked some secretaries to fill out a questionnaire for a study on candy consumption, and as thanks, offered them a nice dish of candy.[68] They asked some of the secretaries to put the dish on their desk and others to put it about six feet away. Each dish had a known number of candies, and every night, the researchers secretly counted how many candies were eaten that day and then refilled the dish to the original amount. When the dish was placed on the desk, the secretaries consumed on average five more chocolates each day, which translates to 125 more calories per day or 2,500 calories a month, which could result in a weight gain of two-thirds of a pound.

Another study about buffets showed that the first food items seen are the ones most selected.[69] In fact, over seventy-five percent of diners selected the first food they saw, and the first three items encountered on the buffet made up two-thirds of all the foods they chose. The researchers suggested that by rearranging food order from healthiest to least healthy, diners will unconsciously choose more of the healthier options.

Stop Cleaning Your Plate. Don't be a member of the Clean Plate Club. When I was in elementary school (around third or fourth grade), I made a decision on my own to eat everything on my lunch plate, even if I didn't like it. I wanted to be healthy and thought this was the best way to do it; needless to say, these were the beginnings of my chunky years. Other people clean their plates for different reasons, and often, the primary one is guilt over wastefulness. Don't feel obligated to eat all of something just because you paid for it. (In other words, don't let that voice inside your head pressure you about all the starving children in Ethiopia that you may have heard about as a kid.)

Sometimes a monster appetite is like an unruly dog in need of training. One of the top five commands in training a dog is the Leave It command. The Leave It command helps you to protect your dog from things that are inappropriate to eat. Sometimes we need to train our appetite to leave it when it's no longer appropriate to eat more. Purposely leaving some predetermined amount of food on your plate each time you eat is one way to train yourself to not clean your plate.

SLOW DOWN

Eating quickly is associated with overeating, excess body weight, being overweight, the incidence of metabolic syndrome, and can cause bloating and flatulence.[70,71,72] It is amazing how we can change the seemingly insignificant factor of eating speed to realize such a widespread positive effect for our life.

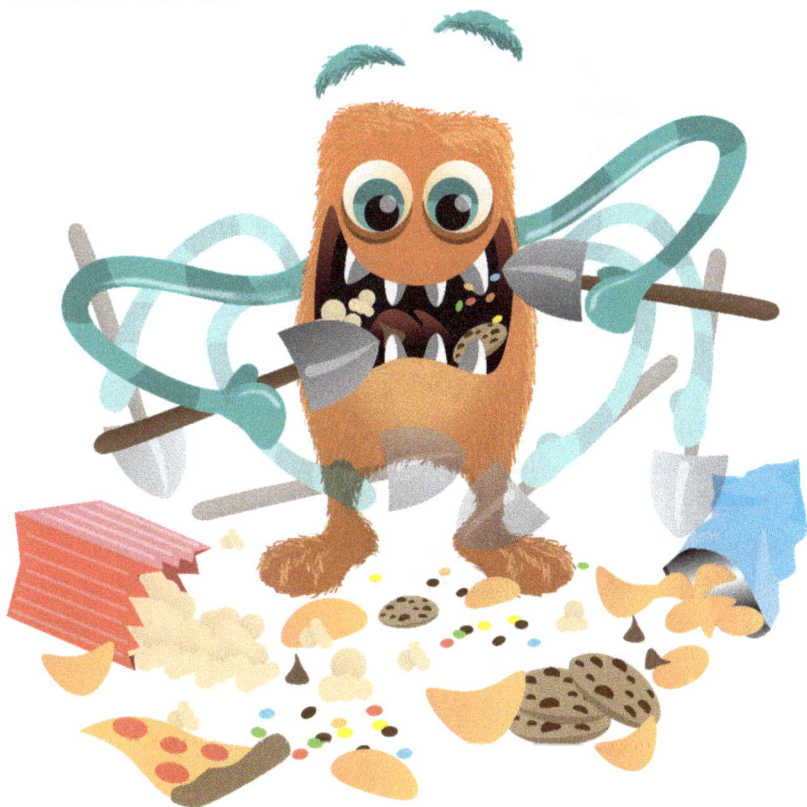

Allow Time for Satiety. According to the Cambridge Dictionary, satiety is "the state of being completely satisfied, especially with food or pleasure, so that you could not have any more."[73] There is a difference between feeling full and feeling satiated (satisfied). Sometimes, we eat quickly and reach fullness, but we continue to eat because we are not yet satisfied. Satiety is not entirely subjective, but it is driven by hormones and physiological processes in the body. Eating fast may hinder the release of these hormones, while eating slower allows the satiety hormones to work effectively. In one study, participants who ate a meal in thirty minutes had higher levels of two peptides that signal satiety than those who are their food in five minutes.[74]

Take Smaller Bites. Research shows that a smaller mouthful of food results in a greater number of chews; therefore, a change in the amount of food we put into our mouth for each bite could be a useful way to control food consumption.[75] I had to teach myself to take smaller bites, and you may need to also. If you are eating chips, break each one into three to five pieces and eat each one separately. I use this to trick my brain into thinking that I'm eating way more chips than I actually am. I rarely eat a whole French fry in one bite, and never by the handfuls anymore. Keep in mind that larger serving bowls and spoons lead to larger portion sizes, and larger portion sizes led to a larger bite sizes. [76] [77] For ways to control portion sizes, see the section *Use Proper Portion Sizes* on page 99. Also, try using smaller eating utensils, because it's harder to load heaps of food onto a smaller fork or spoon.

Don't get caught in the idea that a bigger bite tastes better. It's not true. There is a limit of how much you can taste and adding more food doesn't help. A smaller bite can give just as much flavor in the mouth as a larger one. Personally, the larger amount of food I place into my mouthy each time, the less time I spend chewing and the more food I end up swallowing whole. I've come to the conclusion that when my mouth is full, I can't roll it around and experience all the flavor as well, so I swallow a bunch of it to make room. With a smaller bite, we are able to experience its maximal flavor, like a wine taster who takes sips and not gulps.

Decrease Hand-to-Mouth Speed. When you eat, do your arms resemble the monster's in the picture? Try pausing between bites. You can do this by setting your fork down after each bite, not preparing the next bite while chewing on the current one, not holding the sandwich between bites, and switching hands with each bite (this also exercises you brain when using non-dominant hand).

Preload Your Stomach. No, this does not mean eat appetizers!! Sometimes in restaurants, I will drink an entire glass of water, tea, or coffee while waiting on my food. This helps me in two ways: 1) it kicks off the feeling of fullness and 2) it makes me want to use the restroom before the meal is over and gives me a reason to separate myself from the table before making dessert decisions. (Now, many food experts are in disagreement as to the proper time to drink a beverage during a meal, but I personally opt for before, during, and after—you do what works best for you.) Another way to preload your stomach is to eat first the foods which are lower in energy and larger in volume (i.e., vegetables), while saving the high energy items (aka, the fattening stuff) for the later part of the meal when you are already reaching fullness and satiety.

PLAN THE TIMING OF YOUR MEALS

The body in action is like a symphony. Each organ, hormone, and biochemical pathway acts in conjunction to produce life. Just like in a symphony when it's time for certain instruments to play, our body has processes that are supposed to occur in their correct timing. Eating and sleeping are two very important ones we must take care to keep regular.

Eat at Regular Times. Eating at regular times will prevent hunger storms and other issues like episodes of low blood sugar. When we properly anticipate our meals and plan for regularity, then these problems are eliminated. Use the hunger rating scale on page 55 to estimate when it will be time to eat and to develop a regular eating schedule that works for you. If you know you may have to skip a meal, then pack a healthy meal bar. (Notice, I didn't say candy bar...)

Part of the hunger scale is learning the grades of hunger and how they feel in your own body and then balancing them with the timing for your next meal. At first glance, it may appear that someone should eat before they have reached full hungry; however, this is not the case, and I'm not advocating that someone eat to prevent future hunger. Hunger prevention is something that happens a lot, especially on vacations (i.e., folks may eat extra breakfast because they anticipate skipping lunch, then end up eating lunch too). But what I *am* advocating is eating at the right grade of hunger and establishing a regular meal schedule that works for you.

Reduce Inappropriate Snacking. Some of the reasons we snack include boredom, the presence of snacks, hunger due to poor food choices in the previous meal, and anticipation of future hunger. Late-night snacking is a problem for many people. Consuming the major part of the energy intake at the end of the day is unfavorable on healthy weight balance and may be associated with obesity.[78]

In an interesting study about cravings, participants were prompted by text message to report any cravings, including the item desired, the stength of the craving, and whether they gave in to it. [79] Some of the participants were instructed to play Tetris for three minutes and reported their craving again. The results showed that playing Tetris decreased craving strength for drugs (alcohol, nicotine, caffeine), food and drink, and activities (sex, exercise, gaming). The reason for the effect is unknown but may have something to do with eliminating boredom or inducing distraction. Another interesting study in participants with high degrees of emotional eating showed that food craving was reduced in the smiling group and amplified in the frowning group; so according to this study, we may be able to smile away our cravings.[80]

One way to overcome inappropriate snacking is to use visual cues (just like in the study where participants were trained to choose carrots when they saw a certain picture). I have an elf on a shelf on duty at our house.

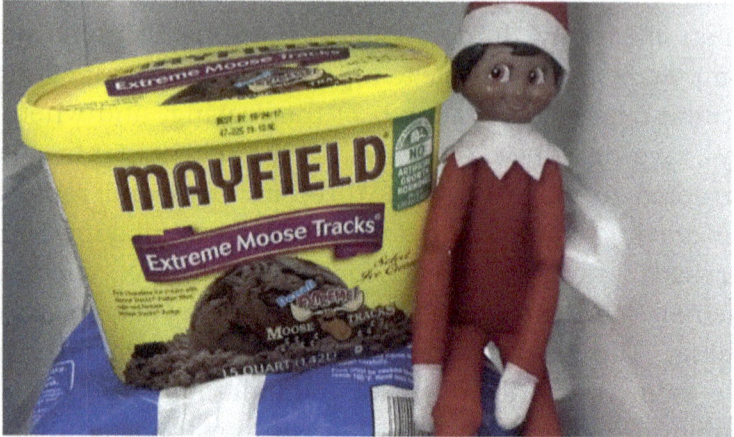

Jennifer Minigh
@jenniferminigh

When you sneak out of bed in the middle of the night and realize #Santa is onto you...

#elfonashelf #holidayproblems

LIMIT RESTAURANT EATING

Up to a third of all the energy we get from food is consumed from restaurants, and a majority of it comes from fast food.[81] Restaurant eating entails bigger portion sizes and higher calorie meals. Research showed that for every single meal a week increase in restaurant eating, BMI was associated with a 0.6 to 0.8 kg/m[2] increase.[82]

Researchers in one study looked at 364 restaurants with food styles ranging across the popular options and measured the energy content of frequently ordered meals.[83] Almost all the meals exceeded typical energy requirements for a single eating occasion. In fact, the meals averaged 1,200 calories, which is over half the recommended daily intake for an adult woman and close to half for an adult man. Meals at three of the four most popular cuisines (American, Italian, and Chinese) averaged closer to 1,500 calories per meal.

Know What You're Getting. It is important to know the caloric quality of food you are getting in a restaurant, especially for women, who risk blowing all their day's calories in one meal. Unfortunately, about half of individual-owned or small-chain restaurants do not provide nutrition information.[84] However, for the ones that do, check out their nutritional menu in advance to determine meals that will work for you. Watch out for calories in disguise that mascaraed as healthy foods. Salads can be some of the highest calorie meals, so pay close attentions. For example, an oriental chicken salad at a popular chain restaurant is 1,390 calories, while a turkey and avocado wrap is 1,260. As an aside... How many people on a diet eat these items and then condemn a person eating a peanut butter milkshake? (By the way, the medium milkshake is 1,060 calories.)

Avoid Buffets. The worst type of restaurant to visit is a buffet. About ninety-two percent of self-served food is eaten.[85] This means when you couple the mentalities of "get my money's worth" with "I'll just have a small bite of everything" that you are likely facing a losing battle at the front line of the buffet. Let's face it—we tend to eat more when there is more variety. Too many things to try, and even a "taste" of something adds up fast. A *bite* of pecan pie at our local buffet is about 70 calories and 3 grams fat. If a person takes about fifty mouthfuls per meal (as research shows on average),[86] then "bites" like this would add up to 3,500 calories for that single meal.

Variety in flavor can affect how much we consume. As we eat a particular food and reach satiety, the pleasure we get from the taste of that food decreases more than for the other foods present.[87] This effect may explain why we grow tired of one item on our plate and then switch our focus to another. Some researchers believe diminished pleasure of food items is a key factor that contributes to the cessation of the meal.[88] If only two or three food items comprise then meal, then it is conceivable to reach satiety sooner than if there were many food items available. Another reason to avoid buffets and limit the variety of foods in a meal.

WATCH OUT FOR HIDDEN CALORIES

Many foods have hidden calories for various reasons. While consumer unawareness is probably the most rampant reason, other reasons include disparity of estimated versus actual nutrition according to the real-life food preparation, as well as deceptive marketing to make foods appear more beneficial than they really are.

Because studies have shown that restaurants often undervalue the actual calorie content of their foods, Dr. Yoni Freedhoff, author of the book *The Diet Fix: Why Diets Fail and How to Make Yours Work*, recommends adding forty percent more calories to non-posted calorie counts for meals at restaurants, and twenty percent more to posted information.[89]

My husband and I had an issue with hidden calories in steamed broccoli we often ate at a local chain restaurant. We were estimating the nutritional information because the restaurant did not post any values for their foods. Over a year later, when they finally did post it, we saw their steamed broccoli was loaded with tons of extra calories and fat. Now, every time we eat at this particular restaurant, he ruminates about at all the times he ate the seemingly heathy vegetable and was duped by restaurant. This "food conspiracy" has become somewhat of a joke in our family as we ponder the possibility of hidden calories in other food establishments and products.

Sauces. Most sauces are butter, oil, cheese, heavy whipping cream, or some thigh-engorging combination of them all. When you are deciding which foods to eat, use the following table to choose the healthiest "flavor" for the dish. For example, if you are having pasta, the lighter sauce would be marinara instead of alfredo. Also, watch out for food descriptions that include "creamy," "cheesy," "sautéed," or "braised in its own juices."

General Nutrition per 2 Tablespoons

	Calories	Fat (grams)	Carbs (grams)	Protein (grams)
SAUCES				
Olive Oil	240	27	0	0
Butter	204	23	0	0.2
Pesto Sauce	160	15	1.5	5.5
Alfredo Sauce	125	12.5	0.8	2.7
Peanut Sauce	86	7.2	3.5	3.6
Duck Sauce	84	5	8.5	0.2
Cheese Sauce	55	4.2	2.2	2.1
Teriyaki Sauce	30	0	5.6	2.1
Sweet and Sour Sauce	28	0	7	0.1
Barbecue	24	0.6	4	0.6
Green Enchilada Sauce	24	2	2	0.4
Marinara	23	0.8	3.5	0.6
Worcestershire Sauce	22	0	6.6	0
DRESSINGS				
Caesar Salad Dressing	160	17	1	1
French Dressing	156	14.2	5	0.3
Ranch Dressing	150	15.5	2	0.3
Bleu Cheese Dressing	150	16	1	0
Thousand Island Dressing	120	11.2	4.6	0.4
Honey Mustard Dressing	100	5.4	14	0.3
Italian Dressing	86	8.2	3	0.1
Balsamic Vinaigrette	60	5	3	0
CONDIMENTS				
Mayonnaise	164	10	7	0.3
Tartar Sauce	150	14.6	4.2	0.3
Ketchup	30	0.1	7.5	0.5
Salsa	8	0.1	2	0.5
Mustard	6	0.3	0.8	0.4
Tabasco Sauce	4	0.2	0.2	0.4

Dressings and Condiments. These items will ring up your calorie bill so fast your head will spin. A typical serving of mayonnaise on a sandwich in restaurant is more than the serving size listed on the nutritional label. I can tell you from experience that when our local sandwich artists are adding mayo to customers' sandwiches, they often squeeze out more than one serving. Other restaurants may even butter your bread before slathering on the mayo—that's almost 400 extra calories right there. Especially with salads, keep a tab on the extra toppings you're getting because cheese, croutons, nuts, and dressing will throw the calorie count past 1,000 before you know it.

When ordering salads and sandwiches, ask to receive dressings and condiments on side. Try dipping your fork in the dressing first, then spear a bite of salad. You'd be surprised how a little dressing actually goes a long way. Another tip is to carry lower calorie condiments with you. Search the internet for a clever way to create single-serve units with straws.

Fancy Coffees and Teas. Coffee and tea minus any additives are basically calorie-free. It's the extra stuff that adds up. One serving of cream is 50 calories and 6 grams of fat. Assuming that you are using the listed serving size of one tablespoon of cream and a teaspoon of sugar (which in all likelihood, you're using much more), then if you drink three to four cups of coffee in a day, you could be consuming an extra 200 to 270 calories and 18 to 24 grams of fat. Doing this every day will add an additional 1,900 of hidden calories to you weekly total. Some designer coffees will cost you more than 500 calories for each cup. For example, a mocha coconut Frappuccino with whipped cream is 710 calories and 26 grams of fat. For the days you need a designer beverage, ask for your coffee or tea to be made "skinny" (i.e., with nonfat or skim milk) and with sugar free flavorings, skip the whipped cream, and stick with the smallest size.

Other Beverages. Alcohol, sodas, and fruit juices all have hidden calories. The average calorie count of a glass of wine, bottle of beer, or can of soda is about 150 calories. The average bottle of wine contains about four glasses of wine, so splitting one during a meal will add 300 calories to the day. Likewise, a can of soda with each meal adds 450 calories. Fruit juices are probably the most deceiving beverage, as most people, believing they are a healthy choice, misjudge the sugar content.

Breaded Foods. Breaded foods are generally fried, and fried foods are very high in calories and fat. Beware of food descriptions such as "crispy" or "crunchy," and try to choose more grilled or baked meats as opposed to breaded and fried ones.

"Healthy" Foods. Fruit juices are not the only "healthy" food substances that can be deceptive. See the sections on *Nutritional Cues* (page 82) and *Fitness Cues* (page 83) for how the food industry appeals to us and diverts our attention away from bad nutritional information. Foods deemed as healthy can have a "halo effect," whereby the food is perceived as being virtuous in all respects and can even impart healthfulness to unhealthy foods. These foods are often eaten without regard to calories (leading to excessive consumption) and paired with unhealthy foods to neutralize or counteract detrimental consequences. For example, adding a side salad to a double cheeseburger or personal pizza may cause people to believe that the overall calorie content of the meal somehow, magically decreases and that the cheeseburger or pizza isn't as destructive to their nutrition plan. The biggest problem with supplemental shakes, smoothies, and energy bars is that they are consumed *in addition to* regular food, *instead of* in place of it.

Consider the hidden calories in dried fruits. Someone who wouldn't consider eating five fresh plums in one setting won't think twice before throwing down a handful of dried ones. The process of drying fruit removes water—not all the calories and other nutrition. Avoid eating heaps of dried fruit, as it is very easy to consume excessive calories in just one snack attack.

Too Small to Matter. Sometimes hidden calorie foods that come in small bits are deemed as too small to count, so they are consumed without consideration. Watch out for things like gum, candy (especially mints or a piece of chocolate here and there), and "a taste of something."

AVOID DESSERT TEMPTATIONS

Everyone is susceptible to temptation...especially to desserts.

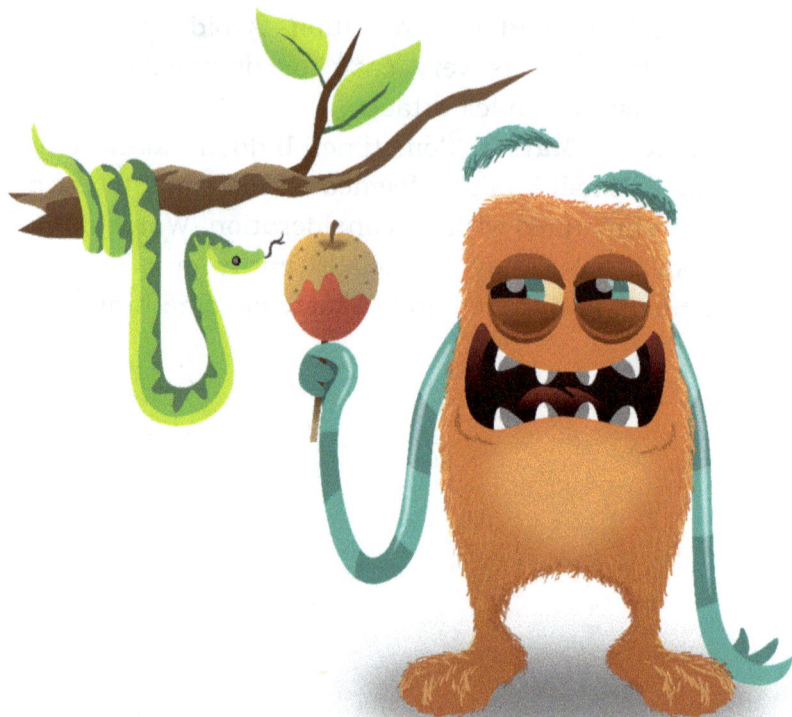

Have a Fallback Alternative. Am I the only one who, after eating a fatty meal, is fixated on dessert despite feeling stuffed? I mean, of all times to deal with intense cravings for something sweet, why does it always seem to happen when I've just made a glutton of myself? Mental coincidence? Perhaps hidden self-destruction? Nope. Looks like there may be some science behind it. Emerging evidence now suggests that the sweet-taste signaling mechanisms in the mouth may influence satiety.[90] There is a popular Italian restaurant that hands out chocolate mint candies after your meal. Perhaps they understand this principle.

If you tend to desire sweet foods after a meal, then come to the meal prepared. Keep some hard candy available to pop in your mouth afterward to satisfy your craving for sweetness.

Take a Break from the Table. While you are enjoying your hard candy, step away from the table for a few minutes to physically relocate yourself away from food. If in a public restaurant, one option is to visit the restroom. Sometime, just being in a restroom is enough to turn off my appetite. While there, you should wash your hands because research shows that wiping one's hands switches the mind's goals,[91] and in terms of eating, it could be used to divert the mind from the goal of eating and allow it to take up a new goal, thus creating a psychological separation from the meal. Personally, I've noticed that when I eat at a rib place where they give you a Wet Wipe, after cleaning my hands with the pungent wipe, I have no desire to eat anymore, so there may be more to this than scientists have uncovered.

DON'T TRUST YOUR INTENTIONS

As humans, we tend to overestimate our good intentions and give ourselves a buy when we fall short, grading our outcome on what should have happened instead of what actually did. In terms of exercise and eating, this phenomenon was demonstrated in a study of normal-weight individuals who were instructed to walk on a treadmill until an undisclosed number of calories was burned and then were asked to estimate how many calories they burned.[92] The group who walked for 200 calories estimated having burned an average of 825 calories—more than four times the actually amount. An hour later, participants were told to eat a meal from a buffet that, in their estimation, would replace the calories they had burned. This same group consumed an average of 825 calories. Not only did the participants overestimate their efforts, their actions fell short of their intentions.

We've all told ourselves that we can go ahead and eat bad today because tomorrow we'll do better. However, research shows that it really doesn't work, because we usually don't compensate for a day's intake by altering the amount consumed on the next day.[93] Our intentions rarely match our actions, and unfortunately, our perceptions of our abilities can be exaggerated.

Instead of relying on our sham intentions for future goodwill, another option is to hold ourselves immediately accountable for our bad choices. Before partaking of something you will later regret, hold it up and make this or a similar declaration out loud: *I declare that I am going to eat this _____ against my better judgment. I understand that I am making this choice out of my own free will and I have a choice to not do it, but I choose to do so anyway despite the circumstances. I take full responsibility for my actions and accept the consequences without complaints or excuses.*

Taming Your Monster Appetite by Jennifer Minigh

Tame Your Tongue

Does your tongue determine which foods you eat? Do you forego healthy foods because they don't taste like chocolate or some other dessert? It's time to tame your tongue and take back control from the appetite monster.

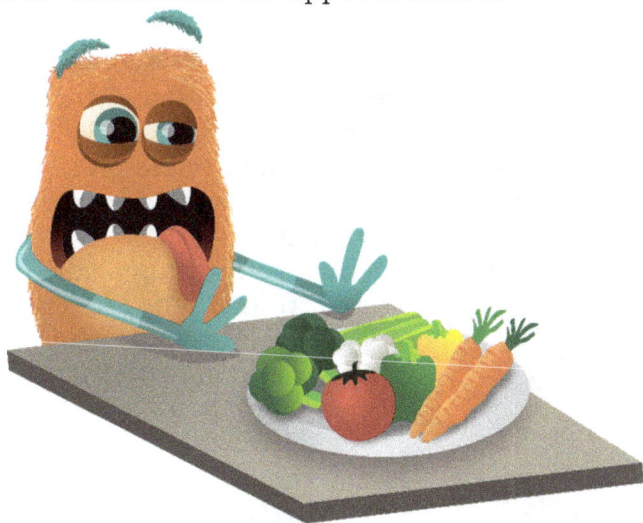

THE SCIENCE OF TASTE

So, what is the purpose of taste, other than allowing us to enjoy food? Many believe the human taste system is a gatekeeper that helps us to consume essential nutrients for survival and to reject potentially harmful or toxic foods.

Although scientists describe seven basic tastes (i.e., bitter, salty, sour, astringent, sweet, pungent, and umami), only five tastes are generally detectable by the tongue. Other flavor descriptions include pungency (i.e., spiciness or hotness), coolness (i.e., fresh or minty), astringency (i.e., puckering like unripe persimmons), and metallic.

The Five Tastes Generally Detectable by the Tongue

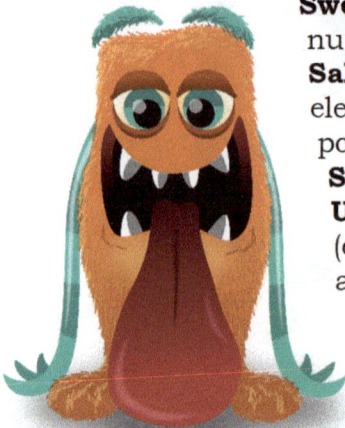

Sweet: indicates energy-rich nutrients

Salty: indicates the presence of electrolytes, such as sodium or potassium

Sour: indicates an acidic food

Umami: the taste of amino acids (e.g., meat broth or aged cheese) and MSG (monosodium glutamate)

Bitter: the most sensitive of the tastes, and is generally perceived as unpleasant, sharp, or disagreeable; many toxins and poisons are bitter

We all have taste preferences. While most people prefer the sweets, others claim spicy foods as their favorite and maintain that these foods produce satiety faster.

It's a cultural phenomenon (especially in the Western world) that foods high in fat *and* carbs are perceived to be the tastiest. Some tastes are prone to induce addiction than others. In rats, high-fat foods,[94] high-sugar foods,[95] and most strongly, combinations of high-fat and high-sugar foods, [96] are candidates for food addiction. In humans, highly processed, tasteful foods are the ones that may have addictive potential.[97]

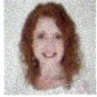

Jennifer Minigh
@jenniferminigh

How can it be that empty calories are so full of flavor?

Taste preference can change under certain circumstances. A reduction in the ability to taste (hypogeusia), loss of taste (ageusia), or a distortion of taste (dysgeusia) can be caused by a dry mouth, minor infections, nutritional deficiencies, injury inside the mouth, use of cigarettes, snuff, or shewing tobacco, certain diseases, and medications. Smell is one of the most prominent influences of taste, and an inability to smell will decrease the ability to taste.

The ability to taste affects the amount we eat. (I can personally attest to this, but many studies prove it too.) However, there is another connection of smell to fat metabolism that researchers don't fully understand yet. In one study, mice that lost their sense of smell were resistant to obesity.[98] Here's what's weird: these smell-deficient mice ate the same high-fat diet as mice that could smell and stayed slim while the smellers grew to twice their normal weight. In addition, the mice with a boosted sense of smell (i.e., super-smellers) got even fatter than the mice with normal abilities to smell. The findings suggest that the aroma of food may play an important role in how the body metabolizes that food.

OUT WITH THE BAD

No matter what our tongue wants, sometimes we need to remove certain influences from it. Do you let your kids hang out with bad influences?

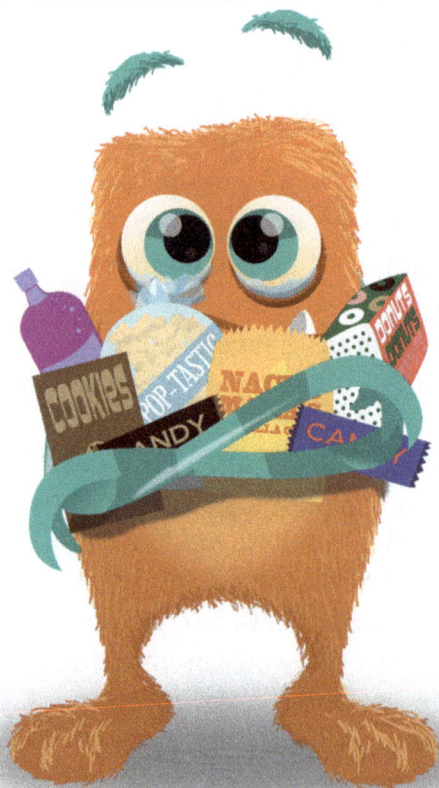

Our daughter loves onions. As a child, she would munch on them like apples. However, when the time of middle school arrived, we had to nix her excessive consumption because we could smell them on her for days.

Is there some food item in your life that needs to go? Or at least to limit the quantity and frequency at which you eat it? Consider making small changes in your lifestyle to eliminate problematic foods. Try choosing one item from the list below and work on it for a month or two until it becomes a natural part of your lifestyle. Don't try to change multiple things at once because this usually leads to frustration and eventual failure. Change your food repertoire *one food at a time.*

Whole Milk

- Use skim milk instead, especially when drinking a glass of milk or using it on cereal.
- If cooking with milk, make half of the amount needed be skim milk.
- Request skim milk in fancy coffee drinks instead of creamer or whole milk.

Butter/Margarine

- For baking, use yogurt, applesauce, or black beans (good for brownies!).
- Use butter substitute sprays. Watch out for the spreads, which are higher in calories and fat. These sprays may require a couple usages before you acquire a taste for them. It generally takes a week and can be speeded up by mixing the bottle well before spraying and allowing the sprayed portion to "breathe" a minute before you eat.

Eggs and Egg Products

- Use egg whites and reduce consumption of yolks. For example, for three scrambled eggs, use two egg whites and one whole egg.
- Use lighter versions of mayonnaise and similar salad dressings.

Beverages

- I never recommend soda, but if you can't quit the high-test stuff cold-turkey, then at least switch to diet.
- Watch out for hidden calories in fancy coffees and teas. Try ordering lower calorie versions.

- Not all fruit juices are the same. At some point, we need to ask ourselves: If something is 10 percent juice and 90 percent sugar water and food coloring, then is it *really* juice? Be sure to read the labels and choose low-sugar versions.

Sweets

- Look for lower calorie or fat options like sugar-free gelatin (low sugar and fat) or angel food cake (low fat).
- Sugar-free hard candy and suckers are great for satisfying an immediate craving for something sweet. Watch out for sugar-free chocolate and caramel candies, because these can have high fat content.
- Opt for fresh fruit instead of cakes or candies. If choosing canned fruit, then make sure you choose fruits in their own juices and not in syrup.

Cheese

- Limit the amount of cheesy pasta you eat.
- Try low-fat or fat-free versions of cheese. You may be amazed how good they can taste. In fact, there is a supermarket brand of fat-free American slices that I prefer over the regular slices every time.
- Avoid cream cheese, but in instances when you need it for a recipe, use the fat-free version, which is surprisingly good.

Fried Foods

- Baking and grilling are better options.
- Air fryers really work, and they give a fried taste without the added fat or calories.
- If you are following the Atkins Diet, don't fall into the trap of eating fried foods.
- Remember that fried vegetables are still fried—and watch out that the "halo" effect of the vegetable does not tempt you into believing that you are eating healthy.

Pizza

- Remove pizza as a weekly meal and try to limit it to once a month.
- Never eat leftovers.
- Don't order extra cheese. Some pizza places will let you request reduced cheese.
- Choose thin crust or hand-tossed instead of deep dish.
- Limit the amount of meat toppings. If a meatless pizza is outside your tolerance, then try to limit yourself to just one kind of meat topping and refrain from getting three or four.

Fast Food

- Try grilled chicken sandwiches instead of burgers.
- Skip the fries.
- In general, hard taco shells are lower in calories than soft ones. Also, use baked shells instead of fried ones.
- Try the salads but watch out for the high calorie and fat dressings.

Foods that have lots of components, like a stuffed burrito, have so many taste components, that if one is left out, the taste change will be minimal; therefore, forego the cheese and sour cream and let the other flavors that were being masked by the cheese and sour cream rise up and fill your palette. Don't be afraid of dropping an ingredient and ruining your meal. Eat and live bravely!

Jennifer Minigh
@jenniferminigh

5-yo boy at the table behind us ordering his burrito:
"And stuff it with the good stuff. You know... the good stuff. ok?"

IN WITH THE GOOD

It's easy to eat healthy foods that taste good, but what about the ones that taste awful?

Have you ever tried baby formula?? It tastes totally disgusting! However, the baby would not agree. In fact, they love the stuff! We can choose to override the displeasure of our tongue. People overlook the tongue's opinion when consuming alcoholic beverages, so it can be done for vegetables too. Acquired taste is a real thing. If babies' can learn to love formula, then you can learn to love new foods, too. Don't be a slave to your tongue. Stop concerning yourself with food that tastes awesome and start learning to appreciate the taste of foods that are good for you.

Just Try It. One of the things our family likes to do is pick out something weird (and healthy) at the grocery store and bring it home for the family to try. We also enjoy visiting the farmers market. Seeing all the fresh produce makes us want to sample new things.

Pick a food that's really good for you, yet you despise the flavor, and train yourself to like it. For example, chose a fruit or vegetable from the *Judging Fruits and Vegetables* and eat at least three bites a day for a few days each week. I did this with raw carrots and by the end of the week, I was enjoying them.

End Pickiness. How many times have I heard parents say their kid will eat only chicken nuggets, pizza, and chips? Where did this pickiness come from?

In most toddlers and preschoolers, erratic appetites with bouts of food neophobia (fear of new foods) and food jags (times of reduced eating) are very common.[99] However, it's the parents' response to these occurrences that shapes the child's eating habits. Research suggests that with time and repeated exposure, most children will accept new foods.[100]

With the exception of the intermittent times of neophobia and food jags, a picky child really isn't picky—they've just had parents who made constant concessions for them. Most of the pickiness in older kids (and adults) is more akin to food snobbishness.

It is absurd to look at an obese ten-year-old eating a bag of chips and drinking a sugar soda and blame that child for his or her bad eating choices. Not only does that child lack understanding in proper eating, but he or she lacks proper discipline from the parents or guardians. As parents, we have the ability to trump our child's decisions. We also have the ability to not purchase or make available to our kids the things that are detrimental to their life and learning. When a child, or even ourselves, refuses to eat anything but junk food, let's not take the easy way out and use pickiness as an excuse to cave in.

Don't Be Afraid to Try. Don't be afraid to try new foods because you don't know how to pronounce or eat it. I remember the first time I encountered queso dip. The server gave each of us a bowlful along with a basket of chips to share. Thinking it was some sort of soup, I ate every bite of mine with a spoon and asked for another bowl. Needless to say, the person sitting across from me was flabbergasted beyond words. Eventually he found the nerve to explain to me what queso was and how to eat it properly. Was I embarrassed? Oh my... However, that wasn't the only time I've done something ridiculous, and I'm sure similar times will come because I refuse to give up on trying new foods.

Recently, my daughter had a similar experience when I made gnocchi for the first time. Dinner comprised sloppy joe sandwiches and a side of buttered gnocchi. Not sure what it was, since I failed to explain it, Julia filled her plate with the gnocchi and covered it with the meat sauce, thinking it was some weird style of pasta. She ate it and never complained until I asked for her opinion of this new food. We got a good laugh over "the worst tasting spaghetti ever."

Julia has always been openminded about trying new foods, even when she was a small child. We used to play the taste game where I would line up things she had never tasted before. Each item varied greatly in flavor and texture. Julia would go down the line, tasting and providing an assessment. She never hesitated to taste new foods because it was adventurous in her mind. As a result, she has never been a picky eater.

Keep Trying. So why did Julia eat "the worst tasting spaghetti ever" if she thought it was bad? Throughout her life, she come to understand that the first taste isn't always telling. She is willing to try something again in the hopes of developing a taste for it. Even when she tried something healthy that she didn't like, we would require her to try it again each year. Our perception of taste changes with age, during and after pregnancy, after medical illnesses or treatments, etc. It is important to give foods another try.

You may remember my story about the "clean plate" time in my elementary life. Because of my decision to eat everything on my plate, even if I didn't like it (and oh how I dreaded celery day), I learned to love lots of different foods that year. There later came a time in my adult life when I needed to increase my daily fiber intake. This was a particularly difficult task, because the taste and texture of the fiber drink activated my gag reflex. Many times, I stood at the sink because I couldn't get a gulp down. I tried everything I could think of to make it work. I even used straws to try to bypass my tongue. After about two weeks of struggling every day to get a glassful down, I began to make some headway. Now, I love the taste and actually look forward to it every morning. It's not unusual for my mouth to water when preparing it. This was the toughest tongue-taming I ever had to do, but it needed to be done.

I hope you never have as much trouble liking a new food as I did with fiber. Just remember that not all foods taste the same under different circumstances. Some foods will taste better to you if they are cold, hot, or room temperature. Don't be afraid to experiment with different temperatures. Likewise, be open to different ways of cooking the item. Something that is grilled will taste different compared to when it's tasted as part of a soup. Everything tastes better when we are in a state of extreme hunger. The next time you fast, consider ending the fast with something you want to acquire a taste for. You will appreciate it so much more.

Eat It Anyway. Did you know that it's okay to eat foods that your tongue doesn't like? Once when David was a poor college student, his only food in the cabinet was a can of green beans and a jar of grape jelly. So, what did he do? He mixed it up and ate it, of course. Here is proof that it is possible to eat something doesn't taste good and live through it, even without emotional scarring.

Water is something many people have an aversion for. Personally, I don't understand how anyone could harbor ill thoughts toward a tasteless refreshing beverage. But it happens. Water is necessary for life and the importance of proper hydration is too comprehensive to be contained in a couple sentences here. Suffice it to say that there are no acceptable excuses for not drinking water on a regular basis (translated as *every* day, *several times* a day). Drinking water is not really a choice of whether you like it or not. It's something that we all must do, so suck it up.

Subdue the Sloth

Hippocrates said: "Eating alone will not keep a man well. He must also take exercise."

This chapter is about another type of appetite—the monster's appetite for laziness.

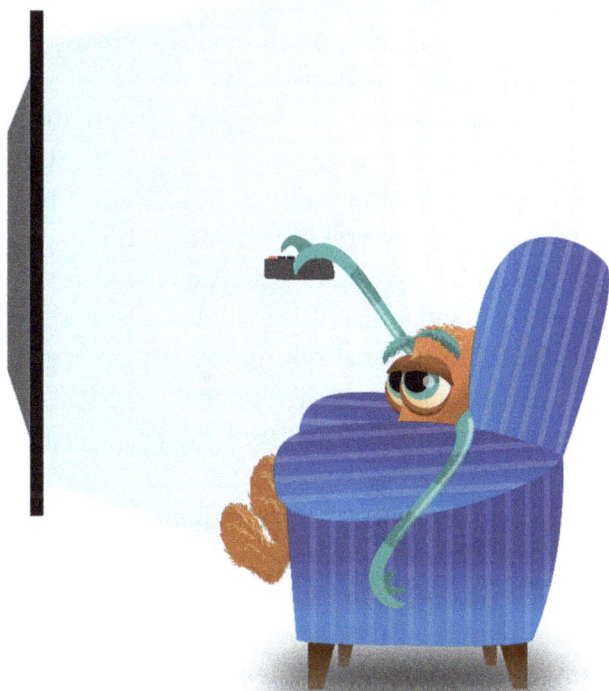

WHAT IS EXERCISE?

The World Health Organization (WHO) defines *physical activity* as:

> *any bodily movement produced by skeletal muscles that requires energy expenditure— including activities undertaken while working, playing, carrying out household chores, traveling, and engaging in recreational pursuits.*

Exercise is a type of physical activity that aims to improve or maintain one's physical fitness. It is measured by the number of calories per body weight a person burns in an hour. One Metabolic Equivalent (MET) is defined as 1 calorie/kg/hour and is roughly equivalent to the energy cost of sitting quietly. Activity that is rated as 1.1 to 2.9 METs is considered to be light-intensity aerobic activity. Moderate intensity is 3.0 to 5.9 METs, and vigorous intensity is 6.0 or more METs. As the MET value goes up, the ability to burn calories does too.

A compendium of physical activities was developed to quantify the energy cost of a wide variety of physical activities from running and biking to vacuuming the floor. See the 2011 Compendium of Physical Activities for a list of activities and their MET value.[101] These values are the ones used by apps like MyFitnessPal to calculate how many calories you burned when exercising. For a rough estimate to calculate the number of calories burned, you can use the formula below. However, this isn't entirely accurate for every single person because everyone's metabolism is different. Also, when entering the time spent doing the activity, use *only* the time spent in movement.

MET value

x

body weight in kilograms

x

time in hours

=

calories burned

When we exercise at a higher intensity, we burn more calories during the activity and also increase the afterburn, which is the burn of calories after the activity stops. This afterburn effect is more officially known as excess post-exercise oxygen consumption, or EPOC for short.

The mechanism for afterburn is still somewhat of a mystery, but it may have something to do with the body using more fat and less carbs after a hard workout, the hormones remaining elevated afterward, or with the body replenishing glycogen stores. Upper body exercise appears to have similar afterburn patterns as lower body exercise.[102]

Research show that afterburn during a three-hour post-exercise period is higher following high-intensity exercise compared with low-intensity exercise. [103] A prolonged afterburn (i.e., three to twenty-four hours after exercise) is achievable; however, the total afterburn amount generally comprises only 6% to 15% of the net energy burn of the exercise,[104] so don't get the misconception that you are burning hundreds of calories an hour after working out. Furthermore, afterburn is unlikely to be prolonged in non-athletic individuals.

EFFECTS OF EXERCISE

The obvious effects of exercise are increased strength, flexibility, and muscle tone, better cardiovascular fitness and endurance, and improved overall health. However, there are so many more benefits that may not be so apparent. Following are just a handful.

> **Jennifer Minigh**
> @jenniferminigh
>
> Every single dose of exercise is 100% effective! Can't say the same thing about meds.
> #health #motivation #fitness

The "Feel-Goods". Anyone who has vigorously performed a sustained strenuous exercise has likely encountered the phenomenon of "runner's high," which is described as a state of euphoria that displaces feelings of pain and fatigue, *making individuals feel like they are invincible and able to work at their maximum potential.* For many years, this experience has been largely attributed to the release of endorphins in the body.

Endorphins are named from the combination of the words "endogenous" (meaning produced within the body) and "morphine." They are opioid-like neurotransmitters that act in your brain to reduce the perception of pain. Endorphins also trigger euphoric feelings.

Recent research has shown that endorphins are not the only chemicals increased in the blood after extreme physical activity. Another neurotransmitter, anandamide, may be responsible for the "runner's high." This chemical can enter the brain to act at cannabinoid receptors (the same receptors that the active ingredient in marijuana acts on). The "feel-goods" may also be attributed to increased levels of serotonin or norepinephrine (neurotransmitters found to be low or depleted in people with depression).

Research continues to show positive effects of exercise on anxiety, stress, and depression. In fact, some evidence suggests that exercise has beneficial effects on depression symptoms that are comparable to those of antidepressant treatments.[105] These positive effects are mediated through both physiological and psychological mechanisms, and they are so powerful that some people can become addicted to exercise. In one study, two groups of runners (one with exercise addiction symptoms and the other without) were deprived of exercise for two weeks.[106] At the end of the withdrawal period, the exercise addiction group showed an increase in depression, confusion, anger, and fatigue.

Better Metabolism. There are three ways your body burns calories:

- *Energy for basic life.* Your basal metabolic rate (BMR) is the amount of energy your body requires to function at complete rest. It's the energy you burn while basically existing, and it represents the minimum amount of energy needed to keep your body alive. Your BMR accounts for up to 75 percent of the energy you burn each day.

- *Energy for digestion.* After you eat, your body turns up the temperature in your digestive system to process the food. This energy accounts for up to ten percent of the energy you burn each day.

- *Energy for physical activity.* This is any energy that is burned when you work out or do any kind of physical movement such as running, vacuuming, brushing your teeth, fidgeting, shivering, etc. The amount of this type of energy you burn each day depends on how active you are.

The higher our BMR, the more calories we can eat every day without gaining weight. More muscle equals a higher BMR, because muscle cells burn more calories than fat cells. For every pound of muscle that you have, your body will burn about 6 calories per day, but for every pound of fat, your body will burn only 2 calories.[107] As we exercise consistently, we increase our muscle mass, which leads to a higher BMR.

Even though both men weigh the same, John can eat almost 300 more calories than James each day, because he has more muscle.

150-pound James With 28% body fat 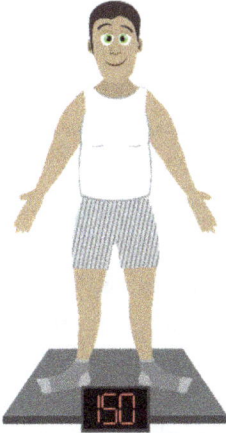	28% body fat means 42 pounds of fat and 108 pounds lean body mass 108 pounds x 13.8 calories/pound means that his **BMR is 1490 calories**
150-pound John With 15% body fat 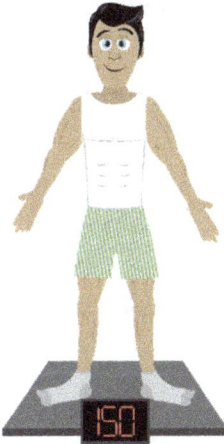	15% body fat means 22.5 pounds of fat) 127.5 pounds x 13.8 calories/pound means that his **BMR is 1760 calories**

You need 13.8 calories to support 1 pound of lean body mass (this includes bone and muscle).

When dieting, it is massively important that the pounds you shed come from fat and not from muscle. So how do you make sure that the weight you lose is fat and not muscle?

During calorie restriction, your body tends to prefer the breakdown of muscle first (it takes fewer calories to break it down). One way to persuade the body to consume stored fat instead is to make it think it needs the muscle. Basically– you'll need to use it or lose it, which means you'll need to increase your daily physical activity. The harder you work your muscles, the more your body will spare them and burn the stored fat instead.

Alleviation of Autoimmune Disease Symptoms. A 2017 review evaluated the clinical evidence regarding the safety, barriers to engagement, and impact of physical activity on autoimmune diseases. [108] In general, the incidences of rheumatoid arthritis, multiple sclerosis, inflammatory bowel diseases, and psoriasis are higher in patients who were engaged in less physical activity.

- In patients with rheumatoid arthritis, those who were physically active during the five years before their formal diagnosis developed a milder disease. Physical activity and exercise improved various aspects of rheumatoid arthritis including joint motility, strength, and functional ability.
- In patients with multiple sclerosis, physical activity was shown to decrease fatigue and to enhance mood, cognitive abilities, and mobility.
- In patients with systemic lupus erythematosus, enhanced quality of life was documented in those who were more physically active.

- Patients with fibromyalgia who were more physically active reported decreased disease severity, reduced pain, and a better quality of life.

Slowing or Reversal of Aging. Aging is closely associated with deterioration of cells and tissues in our body. Research in mice predisposed to accelerated aging showed that five months of endurance exercise resulted in cellular changes that protected against early aging of the mice.[109] In a study of older humans, those participants in the aerobic fitness group had significant increases in brain volume; whereas, the participants in the stretching and toning (nonaerobic) group did not. The researchers concluded that aerobic fitness is important for maintaining and enhancing central nervous system health and cognitive functioning in older adults.[110] In another study of older adults, results showed that aerobic exercise increased the size of the hippocampus, leading to improvements in spatial memory.[111] Specifically, exercise increased the hippocampal volume by 2%, effectively reversing the age-related loss in volume by one to two years.

RECOMMENDED AMOUNT OF EXERCISE

According to the WHO, the recommended levels of physical activity for adults eighteen to sixty-four years old are as follows:[112]

> ...do at least 150 minutes of moderate-intensity aerobic physical activity throughout the week or do at least 75 minutes of vigorous-intensity aerobic physical activity throughout the week or an equivalent combination of moderate- and vigorous-intensity activity.

For additional health benefits, the WHO suggests to either increase the amount of moderate activity to 300 minutes per week, engage in 150 minutes of vigorous activity per week, or some combination thereof. Also, muscle-strengthening activities should be done involving major muscle groups on two or more days a week, and aerobic activity should be performed in bouts of at least ten minutes duration.

"Sitting Is the New Smoking," a catchy slogan that caught on around 2013, increased awareness about how people exercise less and sit more, and the dire health consequences thereof. Since then, the issue has been hotly debated and other terms such as "exercise-deficit disorder" were birthed. One group of researchers defined exercise-deficit disorder as *"reduced levels of moderate-to-vigorous physical activity, inconsistent with public health recommendations."*[113] Regardless of the terminology and theories surrounding the issue, lack of sufficient physical activity is undoubtedly detrimental to one's health.

**NOT here to help you get a *hard* body,
but here to help you get a *lard* body**

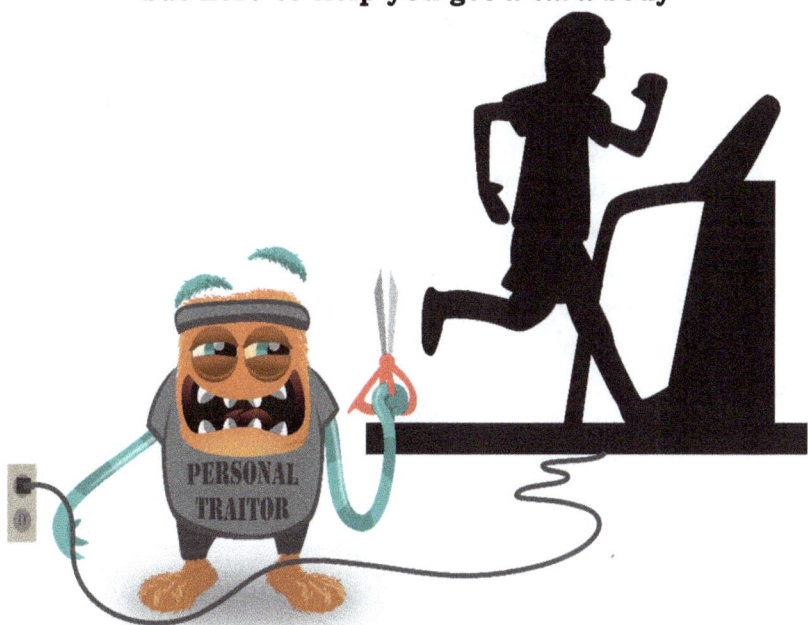

FINDING TIME FOR EXERCISE

Lack of time is the number-one reason people say they don't exercise. Now, we all know there is plenty of time in the day (actually twenty-four hours of it), so why is it that we never have time for things like exercise, but we have time for TV and social media?

Time is not the issue; our perception of it is. When I think of going to work out, I envision the time needed to get dressed, get packed up, get to the gym, get a parking spot, get a workout done, then return home doing all the above in reverse. Wow! That could add up to three hours if not careful. Who has time for that?? Certainly not me!

The truth is—we don't need to join an expensive gym and we don't need fancy workout clothes or equipment. The here and now, with just our body weight, is all we need to get it done. Following are some ways to find time for exercise in your life without completely rearranging it.

Jennifer Minigh
@jenniferminigh

Quit relying on motivation!

Do something because it needs to be done and not because you feel like doing it!

#amwriting #fitness #motivation

In Your Everyday Activities. Burning calories doesn't always have to be done with "exercise." Other everyday activities will burn calories too. The goal is to JUST MOVE and find a way to stay active. Following is a list of activities and the number of calories a 150-pound person would burn doing ten minutes of that activity.

When you do this for 10 minutes...	you could burn this many calories
Carry groceries upstairs	85 calories
Scrub a bathtub	74 calories
Make a bed/change the sheets	38 calories
Paint or wallpaper	38 calories
Wash and wax the car	23 calories
Fidget your feet while sitting	20 calories
Weed the garden	51 calories
Have sex (moderate exertion)	20 calories
Play cards	17 calories
Laugh	11 calories
Kneel in prayer	15 calories
Wash hands, shave, brush teeth, put on makeup	23 calories
March in place	91 calories
Push/pull a stroller	45 calories
Climb stairs slowly	45 calories
Walk a dog	34 calories

Estimates derived from the *2011 Compendium of Physical Activities*[114]

Look for opportunities to move. March in place when brushing your teeth. Take a parking spot in the *back* of the lot instead of driving around for ten minutes looking for a spot by the door. Take the stairs occasionally, even if you need to go up several flights, try to walk at least one of them. When watching TV, stand up and do some squats, push-ups, or sit-ups during the commercial breaks, and by the end of the show, you'll have a good workout accomplished. There are innumerable ways you find ways to increase exercise by just increasing your daily activity level.

Find Ten Minutes. Ten minutes of calisthenics (i.e., squats, push-ups, jumping jacks) a day will burn about 50 extra calories and make your body stronger. Depending on how many ten-minute stints you find a day and how many days a week you do it, you could burn an extra half pound of fat each month. However, the big advantage is immediate mental clarity and focus you will receive after each one.

In Japan, many companies allow their workers to take periodic exercise breaks. During some of these breaks, they even offer communal exercises during which the employees take ten to fifteen minutes to work out together.

Research shows that breaks in sedentary time were associated with better waist circumference, BMI scores, and triglyceride and glucose levels. [115] The Japanese companies have noticed other benefits including improvement in employee morale, camaraderie, and sense of community.

Other countries across the globe are following Japan's lead and offering their employees short exercise breaks throughout the day. Talk to your managers and coworkers about similar opportunities at your workplace. If you work at home, assert your own authority and institute scheduled breaks for yourself.

High-Intensity Activity. According to the WHO, there are multiple ways of accumulating the total of 150 minutes of moderate-intensity activity per week; however, the American College of Sports Medicine recommends that it be thirty minutes per day for five days, and if the intensity is vigorous as opposed to moderate, then twenty minutes on three days.[116] For people who have more demands and restrictions with their free time, the ability to work harder, and not longer, is a wonderful option. The convenience of high-intensity interval training (or commonly referred to as HIIT) is surpassed only by its benefits including improved athletic capacity, cardiovascular fitness, and glucose metabolism.

Even if you don't have twenty minutes for a high-intensity workout, you might be able to find four minutes for a Tabata. A Tabata consists of eight rounds of twenty seconds of work followed by ten seconds of rest. The key is to work at your maximum output during each of those twenty-second intervals.

If you can't find four minutes, then how about one? Carve out some time, no matter how small it may seem— even if it's only a single minute. Take that opportunity and do something intense for one whole time. Make it a game; for example, see how many squats you can do in one minute, then try to beat your best the next time. By just dancing around with jumping jacks, high knees, etc., you'll burn about 10 calories per minute. If you set your alarm to take a single minute every hour, by the end of the day, you could burn over 100 extra calories and you won't have sacrificed a large chuck of time for it.

Finding Time for Fun. Some evidence suggests that the amount of pleasure or displeasure we experience during exercise may influence whether we continue to do it.[117] Furthermore, it is possible that inactivity could stem from previous exercise experiences associated with displeasure. Finding exercises that are fun will increase your desire to find time for it and fortitude to stick with it.

TIMING OF RESULTS

Once upon a time, my aunt decided to grow her own peanuts. She made a planting in a beautiful pot, and not long after, a sprout made its appearance. The plant continued to grow and soon became very large. Meanwhile, her friends who had started their own planting at the same, began bragging on how wonderful their peanuts were. My aunt was discouraged because she saw no such evidence in her own endeavors, but continued to care for the plant, nevertheless, and kept her lack of harvest discreet. Eventually, she reached her limit with their boasting and came clean about her massively beautiful plant that failed to produce. It was only then did she realize that peanuts don't grow on the branches, but are along the roots of the plant, hidden from her view. Turns out, she ended up with a great harvest and a cool story to go along with it.

Because people like instant gratification, exercise can become discouraging if it does not produce fast enough results. However, that does not mean that our toil is in vain. You may not always see immediate fruit for your endeavors, but rest assured that under the surface, things are changing—just like my aunt's peanuts.

Perhaps the hardest result to achieve is the ever-elusive "last ten pounds." It seems to reason that if the last ten pounds are *that hard* to shed, then they will probably be the easiest to regain. Instead of obsessing over them, focus on all the pounds you *did* lose and the health benefits you gained.

You Can Do It!

Mary Shelley, the author of the classic novel *Frankenstein*, wrote, *"I beheld the wretch—the miserable monster whom I had created."* Charles Darwin said, *"We stopped looking for monsters under our bed when we realized that they were inside us."* How did a monster get there? Maybe we ate it...

It's time to deal with the appetite monsters in our life, to get rid of stinkin' thinkin' that plagues our efforts to live a healthier life, and to stop letting these monsters control our thoughts. No more worrying about how or where to start... it's time to take just a single small step of committing to the journey.

Josh, a friend of mine, overhead a guy saying that you get fit at a gym, but you lose weight at the table. This couldn't be truer, and it takes both healthy eating and regular exercise to attain a healthy lifestyle. The world is desperate for an easy fix, but there is none. The search is on for drugs that can mimic the beneficial effects of calorie reduction and exercise without ever having to actually do it. The truth is, real rewards require hard work and commitment.

This book provides an intervention toolbox that not only changes the way you think about food and exercise, but also suggests real doable actions that will help you institute and make those changes manifest in your life. Some of the examples include tips on how to eliminate problematic foods from your food repertoire and add heathy options; how to avoid impulse eating; how to control portion sizes and limiting intake in public settings like restaurants, parties, and work; how to find time for exercise in your busy life; how to recognize intentional marketing and not be affected by it; how to measure the quality of foods, etc.

Lifestyle changes are a process. Our bad habits didn't all form at once, so we will need to address each one separately and in its own time. Also, you may notice new concerns arise as you beat down others. Don't try to battle both, keep working on the one you are addressing, and move to the new one later.

> *"There's a beast in every man, and it stirs when you put a* ~~sword~~ *fork in his hand."*
> *—Jorah Mormont from Game of Thrones*
> *[quote modified]*

Each small problem area in your life that you overcome will have a cumulative effect. The key is to be patient and persistent and not expect miraculous, broad-sweeping changes overnight. Also, don't go it alone. Enlist friends to navigate this lifestyle-change journey with you. Use other tools like social media. Research shows that social media can help people lose weight because individuals are more likely to achieve success with their goals when they make a public commitment to achieving them.[118] Other research shows that we are better equipped to overcome challenging situations when we are close to people we trust. [119] Remember that life can be like a swing—to go higher, we must push against the forces that would hold us down. And having a friend who can push us when we get tired is oh so nice!

Jennifer Minigh
@jenniferminigh

Life can be like a swing... to go higher, sometimes you have to push against the forces that would hold you down
#PressOn #dontgiveup

Once you achieve your lifestyle goals, like reaching your goal weight, it's important to not regress. One researcher examined the medical and scientific literature for the reasons why long-term weight loss was maintained or not.[120] Following is a list of items that contribute to people being able to keep off the weight over time. Focus on strengthening the items on this list to ensure your success.

Self-body perception
Enhanced self-confidence
Social support
Self-motivation
Incentives and rewards
Increased physical activity levels
Healthy eating habits

Following are the barriers people must overcome to maintain the weight loss. Focus on ways to overcome or circumvent the items on this list to prevent any setbacks or failures.

Extreme weather conditions
Natural phenomena (i.e., accidents,
injuries, poor health)
Work commitments
Poor time-management skills
Inability to resist the temptation for food

You are amazing! And don't let anyone, including yourself, ever convince you otherwise. Not only are you ready to embrace the needed lifestyle changes in your life, but you are also armed with tools to make it happen! Stand up and face your appetite monster head on. Get rid of unhealthy behaviors that cause excess weight and inactivity and find a healthy lifestyle you can live with.

Disclaimer:
Before starting any new diet or exercise regime, consult
with your family physician.

Review Request

I hope you have enjoyed this book about how to tame your monster appetite and get rid of the behaviors that cause excess weight and inactivity. If so, then please let other readers know. Let's share the knowledge so that people can find a healthy lifestyle they can live with.

Taming Your Monster Appetite by Jennifer Minigh

About the Author

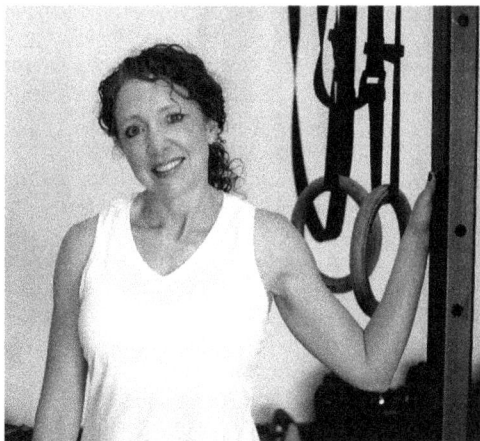

Jennifer Minigh, PhD

Jennifer received her doctorate degree in biomedical science. She has produced over 200 publications in science, medicine, and other genres. In addition, she has worked in the drug industry since 2005 as a regulatory writer for major international pharmaceutical and biotech companies.

Jennifer, her husband David, and her daughter Julia are CrossFit Level 1 trainers. Together, the family enjoys working out, rock climbing, leading a fitness group, and serving in their local church.

Author's Acknowledgements

Thanks to the Lord for blessing my life so abundantly.
Thanks to David and Julia for your love and support.
Thanks to Heather May, Shelby Petitt, and Josh Hickey for sharing your artistic gifts.
Thanks to Chase Dixon for being my handsome cover model.
Thanks to all my friends and family for putting up with my incessant prattle about nutrition and exercise.
Thanks to the RP Fitness crew for your acceptance and love.

References & Resources

[1] Ruddock HK, Dickson JM, Field M, Hardman CA. Eating to live or living to eat? Exploring the causal attributions of self-perceived food addiction. *Appetite*. 2015;95:262–68.

[2] Kraschnewski JL, Boan J, Esposito J, Sherwood NE, Lehman EB, Kephart DK, Sciamanna CN. Long-term weight loss maintenance in the United States. *Int J Obes (Lond)*. 2010;34:1644–54.

[3] Anderson JW, Konz EC, Frederich RC, Wood CL. Long-term weight-loss maintenance: a meta-analysis of U.S. studies. *Am J Clin Nutr*. 2001;74:579–84.

[4] Weiss EC, Galuska DA, Kettel Khan L, Gillespie C, Serdula MK. Weight regain in U.S. adults who experienced substantial weight loss, 1999–2002. *Am J Prev Med*. 2007;33:34–40.

[5] "Lose Weight by Focusing on Mental Health First." Orlando Health. Accessed June 21, 2017. http://oh.multimedia-newsroom.com/index.php/2015/12/01/lose-weight-by-focusing-on-mental-health-first/.

[6] Proverbs 23:7.

[7] Hölzel BK, Carmody J, Vangel M, Congleton C, Yerramsetti SM, Gard T, Lazar SW. Mindfulness practice leads to increases in regional brain gray matter density. *Psychiatry Res*. 2011;191(1):36–43.

[8] Bezzola L1, Mérillat S, Gaser C, Jäncke L. Training-induced neural plasticity in golf novices. *J Neurosci*. 2011;31(35):12444–8.

[9] Vernon B, Nelson E. Exposure to suggestion and creation of false auditory memories. *Psychol Rep*. 2000;86(1):344–6.

[10] Nakata R, Kawai N. The "social" facilitation of eating without the presence of others: Self-reflection on eating makes food taste better and people eat more. *Physiol Behav*. 2017;179:23–9.

[11] Centers for Disease Control and Prevention. "Physical fitness" in the glossary of terms. www.cdc.gov/physicalactivity/basics/glossary/index.htm, accessed June 20, 2017.

[12] Lally P, van Jaarsveld CHM, Potts HWW, Wardle J. How are habits formed: modelling habit formation in the real world. *Euro J Soc Psychol*. 2010;40:998–1009.

[13] Lally P, Wardle J, Gardner B. Experiences of habit formation: A qualitative study. *Psych Health & Med*. 2011;16(4):484–9.

[14] Mötteli S, Keller C, Siegrist M, Barbey J, Bucher T. Consumers' practical understanding of healthy food choices: a fake food experiment. *Br J Nutr*. 2016;116(3):559–66.

[15] Kakoschke N, Kemps E, Tiggemann M. Attentional bias modification encourages healthy eating. *Eat Behav*. 2014;15(1):120–4.

16 Lin PY, Wood W, Monterosso J. Healthy eating habits protect against temptations. *Appetite.* 2016;103:432–40.

17 Cordain L, Lindeberg S, Hurtado M, et al. Acne vulgaris: a disease of Western civilization. *Arch Dermatol.* 2002;138(12):1584–90.

18 "Preventing Chronic Disease | Defining Powerhouse Fruits and Vegetables: A Nutrient Density Approach - CDC." Centers for Disease Control and Prevention. June 05, 2014. https://www.cdc.gov/pcd/issues/2014/13_0390.htm. Accessed July 11, 2017.

19 Foster-Powell K, Holt SH, Brand-Miller JC. International table of glycemic index and glycemic load values: 2002. *Am J Clin Nutr.* 2002 Jul;76(1):5–56.

20 Magnuson BA, Burdock GA, Doull J. Aspartame: a safety evaluation based on current use levels, regulations, and toxicological and epidemiological studies. *Crit Rev Toxicol.* 2007;37:629–727.

21 M D Reuber. Carcinogenicity of saccharin. *Environ Health Perspect.* 1978; 25: 173–200.

22 Ominchanski, L. "You Count, Calories Don't." 1992. https://medical.mit.edu/sites/default/files/hunger_scale.pdf. Accessed July 13, 2017.

23 Di Noia, J. "Preventing Chronic Disease | Defining Powerhouse Fruits and Vegetables: A Nutrient Density Approach—CDC." Centers for Disease Control and Prevention. June 05, 2014. https://www.cdc.gov/pcd/issues/2014/13_0390.htm. Accessed January 08, 2018.

24 Redbook, and Marygrace Taylor. "The Best Apps for Food Journaling." RedbookMag.com. May 15, 2017. http://www.redbookmag.com/body/healthy-eating/advice/g614/lose-weight-apps-tools/. Accessed July 14, 2017.

25 Proverbs 9:17 New International Version

26 Young LR, Nestle M. The contribution of expanding portion sizes to the US obesity epidemic. *Am J Public Health.* 2002;92:246–9.

27 Marchiori D1, Corneille O, Klein O.Container size influences snack food intake independently of portion size. *Appetite.* 2012 Jun;58(3):814 7.

28 Wansink B, Kim J. Bad popcorn in big buckets: portion size can influence intake as much as taste. *J Nutr Educ Behav.* 2005;37(5):242–5.

29 Antonuk B1, Block LG. The effect of single serving versus entire package nutritional information on consumption norms and actual consumption of a snack food. *J Nutr Educ Behav.* 2006;38(6):365–70.

30 "Stomach." The Columbia Encyclopedia, 6th ed. http://www.encyclopedia.com/medicine/anatomy-and-

physiology/anatomy-and-physiology/stomach. Accessed July 25, 2017.

31 Li XE, Jervis SM, Drake MA. Examining extrinsic factors that influence product acceptance: a review. *J Food Sci.* 2015;80(5):R901–9.

32 Ryan S. Elder, Ann E. Schlosser, Morgan Poor, Lidan Xu. So Close I Can Almost Sense It: The Interplay between Sensory Imagery and Psychological Distance. *J Consumer Res.* 2017; 4(4):877–94.

33 Papies EK1. Tempting food words activate eating simulations. *Front Psychol.* 2013;4:838.

34 Topolinski S, Boecker L. Mouth-watering words: Articulatory inductions of eating-like mouth movements increase perceived food palatability. *Appetite.* 2016;99:112–20.

35 Zhong CB, Devoe SE. You are how you eat: fast food and impatience. *Psychol Sci.* 2010;21(5):619–22.

36 Martínez Steele E, Popkin BM, Swinburn B, Monteiro CA. The share of ultra-processed foods and the overall nutritional quality of diets in the US: evidence from a nationally representative cross-sectional study. *Popul Health Metr.* 2017;15(1):6.

37 Gilston A, Privitera GJ. A "healthy" color: information about healthy eating attenuates the "red effect". *Glob J Health Sci.* 2015;8(1):56–61.

38 Walsh LM, Toma RB, Tuveson RV, Sondhi L. Color preference and food choice among children. *J Psychol.* 1990;124(6):645–53.

39 Wąsowicz G, Styśko-Kunkowska M, Grunert KG. The meaning of colours in nutrition labelling in the context of expert and consumer criteria of evaluating food product healthfulness. *J Health Psychol.* 2015;20(6):907–20.

40 Levitan CA, Zampini M, Li R, Spence C. Assessing the role of color cues and people's beliefs about color-flavor associations on the discrimination of the flavor of sugar-coated chocolates. *Chem Senses.* 2008;33(5):415–23.

41 Enax L, Weber B, Ahlers M, et al. Food packaging cues influence taste perception and increase effort provision for a recommended snack product in children. *Front Psychol.* 2015;6:882.

42 Lapierre MA, Vaala SE, Linebarger DL. Influence of licensed spokescharacters and health cues on children's ratings of cereal taste. *Arch Pediatr Adolesc Med.* 2011;165(3):229–34.

43 Lapierre MA, Brown AM, Houtzer HV, Thomas TJ. Child-directed and nutrition-focused marketing cues on food packaging: links to nutritional content. *Public Health Nutr.* 2017;20(5):765–73.

44 Colby SE, Johnson L, Scheett A, Hoverson B. Nutrition marketing on food labels. *J Nutr Educ Behav.* 2010;42(2):92–8.

45 Walters A, Long M. The effect of food label cues on perceptions of quality and purchase intentions among high-involvement consumers

with varying levels of nutrition knowledge. *J Nutr Educ Behav.* 2012;44(4):350–4.

[46] Koenigstorfer J, Groeppel-Klein A, Kettenbaum M, Klicker K. Eat fit. Get big? How fitness cues influence food consumption volumes. *Appetite.* 2013;65:165–9.

[47] Center for Food Safety and Applied Nutrition. "Labeling & Nutrition - Guidance for Industry: Trans Fatty Acids in Nutrition Labeling, Nutrient Content Claims, Health Claims; Small Entity Compliance Guide." U S Food and Drug Administration Home Page. https://www.fda.gov/food/guidanceregulation/guidancedocumentsr egulatoryinformation/labelingnutrition/ucm053479.htm. Accessed July 13, 2017.

[48] Gustat J, Lee YS, O'Malley K, Luckett B, Myers L, Terrell L, Amoss L, Fitzgerald E, Stevenson PT, Johnson CC. Personal characteristics, cooking at home and shopping frequency influence consumption. *Prev Med Rep.* 2017;6:104–10.

[49] Minaker LM, Olstad DL, Thompson ME, et al. Associations between frequency of food shopping at different store types and diet and weight outcomes: findings from the NEWPATH study. *Public Health Nutr.* 2016;19(12):2268–77.

[50] Deighton K, Duckworth L, Matu J, et al. Mouth rinsing with a sweet solution increases energy expenditure and decreases appetite during 60 min of self-regulated walking exercise. *Appl Physiol Nutr Metab.* 2016;41(12):1255–61.

[51] Todd JE. Changes in consumption of food away from home and intakes of energy and other nutrients among US working-age adults, 2005-2014. *Public Health Nutr.* 2017;20(18):3238–46.

[52] Scully P, Reid O, Macken A, et al. Food and beverage cues in UK and Irish children-television programming. *Arch Dis Child.* 2014;99(11):979–84.

[53] Passamonti JB, Rowe C, Schwarzbauer MP, et al. Personality predicts the brain's response to viewing appetizing foods: The neural basis of a risk factor for overeating. *J Neurosci.* 2009;29(1):43–51.

[54] "Ready, steady, look." Ready, steady, look - Epicure. http://www.theage.com.au/articles/2004/03/01/1077989479310. html. Accessed January 08, 2018.

[55] de Solier I. TV dinners: Culinary television, education and distinction. *Continuum: J Media & Cultural Studies.* 2005;19:465–81.

[56] Prince, 2014. How we're fed 434 hours of TV cookery a week—But the more they show, the less we cook. Daily Mail Online, 26th September. http://www.dailymail.co.uk/tvshowbiz/article-2771553/How-fed-434-hours-TV-cookery-week-cook.html. Accessed January 4, 2017.

[57] Ray K. Domesticating cuisine: Food and aesthetics on American television. *Gastronomica*. 2007;7:50–63.

[58] Pope L, Latimer L, Wansink B. Viewers vs. doers: The relationship between watching food television and BMI. *Appetite*. 2015;90:131-135.

[59] Bodenlos JS, Wormuth BM. Watching a food-related television show and caloric intake. A laboratory study. *Appetite*. 2013;61:8–12.

[60] Pope L, Latimer L, Wansink B. Viewers vs. doers. The relationship between watching food television and BMI. *Appetite*. 2015;90:131-5.

[61] Wikipedia contributors, "Food porn," *Wikipedia, The Free Encyclopedia*, https://en.wikipedia.org/w/index.php?title=Food_porn&oldid=8035 68173. Accessed December 3, 2017.

[62] Abbar, S., Mejova, Y., & Weber, I. (2015). You Tweet what you eat: Studying food consumption through Twitter. Paper presented at CHI 2015, April 18–23, Seoul, Republic of Korea.

[63] Lock C, Brindal E, Hendrie GA, Cox DN. Contextual and environmental influences on reported dietary energy intake at evening eating occasions. *Eat Behav*. 2016;21:155–60.

[64] Hermans RC, Larsen JK, Herman CP, Engels RC. How much should I eat? Situational norms affect young women's food intake during meal time. *Br J Nutr*. 2012;107(4):588–94.

[65] Almiron-Roig E, Tsiountsioura M, Lewis HB, Wu J, Solis-Trapala I, Jebb SA. Large portion sizes increase bite size and eating rate in overweight women. *Physiol Behav*. 2015;139:297–302.

[66] van Kleef E1, Shimizu M, Wansink B. Serving bowl selection biases the amount of food served. *J Nutr Educ Behav*. 2012;44(1):66–70.

[67] Bates KJ1, Byker Shanks C2. Placement of a take-out container during meal influences energy intake. *Eat Behav*. 2015;19:181-3.

[68] Wansink B, Painter JE, Lee YK. The office candy dish: proximity's influence on estimated and actual consumption. *Int J Obes (Lond)*. 2006;30:871–5.

[69] Wansink B, Hanks AS. Slim by design: serving healthy foods first in buffet lines improves overall meal selection. *PLoS One*. 2013;8(10):e77055.

[70] Ohkuma T, Hirakawa Y, Nakamura U, Kiyohara Y, Kitazono T, Ninomiya T. Association between eating rate and obesity: a systematic review and meta-analysis. *Int J Obes* (Lond). 2015;39(11):1589–96.

[71] Maruyama K, Sato S, Ohira T, et al. The joint impact on being overweight of self reported behaviours of eating quickly and eating until full: cross sectional survey. *BMJ*. 2008;337:a2002.

[72] Zhu B, Haruyama Y, Muto T, Yamazaki T. Association between eating speed and metabolic syndrome in a three-year population-based cohort study. *J Epidemiol*. 2015;25(4):332–6.

73 Definition of "satiety" from the Cambridge Advanced Learner's Dictionary & Thesaurus © Cambridge University Press.

74 Kokkinos A, le Roux CW, Alexiadou K, et al. Eating slowly increases the postprandial response of the anorexigenic gut hormones, peptide YY and glucagon-like peptide-1. *J Clin Endocrinol Metab.* 2010;95(1):333–7.

75 Goto T, Nakamich A, Watanabe M, Nagao K, Matsuyama M, Ichikawa T. Influence of food volume per mouthful on chewing and bolus properties. *Physiol Behav.* 2015;141:58–62.

76 Wansink B, van Ittersum K, Painter JE. Ice cream illusions bowls, spoons, and self-served portion sizes. *Am J Prev Med.* 2006;31(3):240–3.

77 Almiron-Roig E, Tsiountsioura M, Lewis HB, Wu J, Solis-Trapala I, Jebb SA. Large portion sizes increase bite size and eating rate in overweight women. *Physiol Behav.* 2015;139:297–302.

78 Berg C, Forslund HB. The influence of portion size and timing of meals on weight balance and obesity. *Curr Obes Rep.* 2015;4(1):11–8.

79 Skorka-Brown J, Andrade J, Whalley B, May J. Playing Tetris decreases drug and other cravings in real world settings. *Addict Behav.* 2015;51:165–70.

80 Schmidt J, Martin A. Smile away your cravings—facial feedback modulates cue-induced food cravings. *Appetite.* 2017;116:536–43.

81 Todd JE. Changes in consumption of food away from home and intakes of energy and other nutrients among US working-age adults, 2005-2014. *Public Health Nutr.* 2017;20(18):3238–46.

82 Bhutani S, Schoeller DA, Walsh MC, McWilliams C. Frequency of Eating Out at Both Fast-Food and Sit-Down Restaurants Was Associated With High Body Mass Index in Non-Large Metropolitan Communities in Midwest. *Am J Health Promot.* 2016;0890117116660772.

83 Urban LE, Weber JL, Heyman MB, et al. Energy Contents of Frequently Ordered Restaurant Meals and Comparison with Human Energy Requirements and U.S. Department of Agriculture Database Information: A Multisite Randomized Study. *J Acad Nutr Diet.* 2016;116(4):590–8.

84 Urban LE, Weber JL, Heyman MB, et al. Energy Contents of Frequently Ordered Restaurant Meals and Comparison with Human Energy Requirements and U.S. Department of Agriculture Database Information: A Multisite Randomized Study. *J Acad Nutr Diet.* 2016;116(4):590–8.

85 Wansink B, Johnson KA. The clean plate club: about 92% of self-served food is eaten. *Int J Obes (Lond).* 2015;39(2):371–4.

[86] Ioakimidis I1, Zandian M, Eriksson-Marklund L, Bergh C, Grigoriadis A, Södersten P. Description of chewing and food intake over the course of a meal. *Physiol Behav.* 2011;104(5):761–9.

[87] Rolls BJ, Rolls ET, Rowe EA, Sweeney K. Sensory specific satiety in man. *Physiol Behav.* 1981;27:137–42.

[88] Sørensen LB, Møller P, Flint A., Martens M, Raben A. Effect of sensory perception of foods on appetite and food intake: A review of studies on humans. *Int J Obes.* 2003;27:1152–66.

[89] Belluz, Julia. "The right way to count calories, according to weight loss experts." Vox. December 03, 2014. https://www.vox.com/2014/12/3/7324047/how-to-count-calories. Accessed December 21, 2017.

[90] Beglinger C., Degen L. Gastrointestinal satiety signals in humans— Physiologic roles for GLP-1 and PYY? *Physiol Behav.* 2006;89:460–4.

[91] Dong P, Lee SW. Embodiment as procedures: Physical cleansing changes goal priming effects. *J Exp Psychol Gen.* 2017;146(4):592– 605.

[92] Willbond SM, Laviolette MA, Duval K, Doucet E. Normal weight men and women overestimate exercise energy expenditure. *J Sports Med Phys Fitness.* 2010;50(4):377–84.

[93] Levitsky DA, Raea Limb JE, Wilkinson L, Sewall A, Zhong Y, Olabi A, Hunter J. Lack of negative autocorrelations of daily food intake on successive days challenges the concept of the regulation of body weight in humans. *Appetite.* 2017;116:277–83.

[94] Bocarsly ME, Berner LA, Hoebel BG, Avena NM. Rats that binge eat fat-rich food do not show somatic signs or anxiety associated with opiate-like withdrawal: implications for nutrient-specific food addiction behaviors. *Physiol Behav.* 2011;104:865–72.

[95] Avena NM, Rada P, Hoebel BG. Evidence for sugar addiction: behavioral and neurochemical effects of intermittent, excessive sugar intake. *Neurosci Biobehav Rev.* 2008;32:20–39.

[96] Johnson PM, Kenny PJ. Dopamine D2 receptors in addiction-like reward dysfunction and compulsive eating in obese rats. *Nat Neurosci.* 2010;13:635–41.

[97] Gearhardt A, Davis C, Kuschner R, Brownell K. The addiction potential of hyperpalatable foods. *Curr Drug Abuse Rev.* 2011;4:140– 5.

[98] Riera CE, Tsaousidou E, Halloran J, et al. The sense of smell impacts metabolic health and obesity. *Cell Metab.* 2017;26(1):198–211.

[99] Dovey TM, Staples PA, Gibson EL, Halford JC. Food neophobia and 'picky/fussy' eating in children: a review. *Appetite.* 2008;50:181–93.

[100] Birch LL, Marlin DW. I don't like it; I never tried it: effects of exposure on two-year-old children's food preferences. *Appetite.* 1982;3:353–60.

[101] Ainsworth BE, Haskell WL, Herrmann SD, et al. 2011 Compendium of Physical Activities: a second update of codes and MET values. *Med Sci Sports Exerc.* 2011;43(8):1575–81.

[102] Short KR, Wiest JM, Sedlock DA. The effect of upper body exercise intensity and duration on post-exercise oxygen consumption. *Int J Sports Med.* 1996;17(8):559–63.

[103] Phelain JF, Reinke E, Harris MA, Melby CL. Postexercise energy expenditure and substrate oxidation in young women resulting from exercise bouts of different intensity. *J Am Coll Nutr.* 1997;16(2):140–6.

[104] LaForgia J, Withers RT, Gore CJ. Effects of exercise intensity and duration on the excess post-exercise oxygen consumption. *J Sports Sci.* 2006;24(12):1247–64.

[105] Dinas PC, Koutedakis Y, Flouris AD. Effects of exercise and physical activity on depression. *Ir J Med Sci.* 2011;180(2):319–25.

[106] Antunes HK, Leite GS, Lee KS, et al. Exercise deprivation increases negative mood in exercise-addicted subjects and modifies their biochemical markers. *Physiol Behav.* 2016;156:182–90.

[107] Wang Z, Heshka S, Zhang K, Boozer CN, Heymsfield SB. Resting energy expenditure: systematic organization and critique of prediction methods. *Obesity Research.* 2001;9:331–6.

[108] Sharif K, Watad A, Bragazzi NL, Lichtbroun M3 Amital H, Shoenfeld Y. Physical activity and autoimmune diseases: Get moving and manage the disease. *Autoimmun Rev.* 201;17(1):53–72.

[109] Safdar A, Bourgeois JM, Ogborn DI, et al. Endurance exercise rescues progeroid aging and induces systemic mitochondrial rejuvenation in mtDNA mutator mice. *Proc Natl Acad Sci USA.* 2011;108(10):4135–40.

[110] Colcombe SJ, Erickson KI, Scalf PE, et al. Aerobic exercise training increases brain volume in aging humans. *J Gerontol A Biol Sci Med Sci.* 2006;61(11):1166–70.

[111] Erickson KI, Voss MW, Prakash RS, et al. Exercise training increases size of hippocampus and improves memory. *Proc Natl Acad Sci USA.* 2011;108(7):3017–22.

[112] "Global Strategy on Diet, Physical Activity and Health: Physical Activity and Adults." WHO. http://www.who.int/dietphysicalactivity/factsheet_adults/en/. Accessed December 27, 2017.

[113] Stracciolini A, Myer GD, Faigenbaum AD. Exercise-deficit disorder in children: are we ready to make this diagnosis? *Phys Sportsmed.* 2013;41(1):94–101.

[114] Ainsworth BE, Haskell WL, Herrmann SD, Meckes N, Bassett DR Jr, Tudor-Locke C, Greer JL, Vezina J, et al. 2011 Compendium of

Physical Activities: a second update of codes and MET values. *Med Sci Sports Exerc.* 2011;43(8):1575–81.

[115] Healy GN, Dunstan DW, Salmon J, et al. Breaks in sedentary time: beneficial associations with metabolic risk. *Diabetes Care.* 2008;31(4):661–6.

[116] Garber CE, Blissmer B, Deschenes MR, et al. American College of Sports Medicine position stand. Quantity and quality of exercise for developing and maintaining cardiorespiratory, musculoskeletal, and neuromotor fitness in apparently healthy adults: guidance for prescribing exercise. *Med Sci Sports Exerc.* 2011;43(7):1334–59.

[117] Ekkekakis P. People have feelings! Exercise psychology in paradigmatic transition. *Curr Opin Psychol.* 2017;16:84–8.

[118] Bradford TW, Grier SA, Henderson GR. Weight loss through virtual support communities: a role for identity-based motivation in public commitment. *J Interactive Market.* 2017;40:9.

[119] Lougheed JP, Koval P, Hollenstein T. Sharing the burden: the interpersonal regulation of emotional arousal in mother-daughter dyads. *Emotion.* 2016;16(1):83–93.

[120] Gupta H. Barriers to and facilitators of long term weight loss maintenance in adult UK people: a thematic analysis. *Int J Prev Med.* 2014;5(12):1512–20.